Advanced Drug Delivery Systems - Innovations in Nanoparticles, Biopolymers, and Natural Extracts

Edited by Brajesh Kumar

Published in London, United Kingdom

Advanced Drug Delivery Systems - Innovations in Nanoparticles, Biopolymers, and Natural Extracts
http://dx.doi.org/10.5772/intechopen.1006011
Edited by Brajesh Kumar

Contributors
Aakif Khan, Abdullah All Mamun Bhuiyan, Anupriya D'Souza, Awatef Alshehri, Faisal Khan, Giulia Bennici, I. Helen Diana, Lubna Alhudhali, Maram Almohaywi, Mariusz Jaremko, Mawadda Alghrably, Mohammad Borhan Uddin, Numan Fazal, Raghuvir Pissurlenkar, Ratin Al Samir, Samah Al-Harthi, Vanathi Sundarapandiyan, Zia Ur Rahman, Łukasz Jaremko

First published in London, United Kingdom, 2025 by IntechOpen
IntechOpen is the global imprint of INTECHOPEN LIMITED, registered in England and Wales, registration number: 11086078, 167-169 Great Portland Street, London, W1W 5PF, United Kingdom

For EU product safety concerns: IN TECH d.o.o., Prolaz Marije Krucifikse Kozulić 3, 51000 Rijeka, Croatia, info@intechopen.com or visit our website at intechopen.com.

British Library Cataloguing-in-Publication Data
A catalogue record for this book is available from the British Library

Advanced Drug Delivery Systems - Innovations in Nanoparticles, Biopolymers, and Natural Extracts
Edited by Brajesh Kumar
p. cm.
Print ISBN 978-1-83634-899-3
Online ISBN 978-1-83634-898-6
eBook (PDF) ISBN 978-1-83634-900-6

Meet the editor

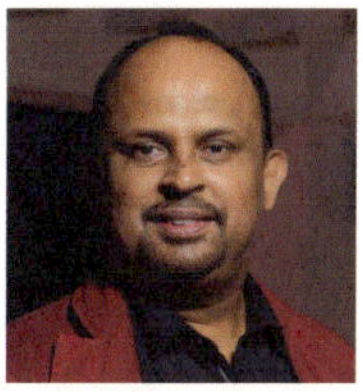

Dr. Brajesh Kumar is an Assistant Professor and the Head of the Department of Chemistry at TATA College, Kolhan University, Chaibasa, India. He received a Ph.D. in Chemistry from the University of Delhi, India, in 2009. He is a pioneering researcher in green chemistry, nanosynthesis, environmental remediation, photocatalysis, nanomedicine, and polymer and natural product extraction. Dr. Kumar has several national and international fellowships to his credit and has worked as a faculty member at various universities throughout India, Ecuador, and South Korea. He holds two registered patents and is a member of the American Chemical Society, the Indian Science Congress Association (ISCA), and the Indian Society of Chemists and Biologists (ISCB). He has published more than 90 research articles (h-index 40, citations > 5140) and is an active reviewer for more than 70 journals. He was also listed among the World's Top 2% of Scientists by Stanford University, USA, in 2021, 2022, 2023, and 2024.

Contents

Preface

This Edited Volume is a collection of reviewed and relevant research chapters on developments in drug delivery systems. The book includes scholarly contributions from various authors and is edited by a group of experts in the field. Each contribution comes as a separate chapter complete in itself but directly related to the book's topics and objectives.

The book contains five chapters:

1. pH-Sensitive Carbonate Apatite Nanoparticles Facilitate the Delivery of siRNA in Breast Cancer Cells

2. Albumin as a Drug Delivery System: Mechanisms, Applications, and Innovations

3. Nanoparticle-Loaded In-Situ Gels: A Paradigm Shift in Ophthalmic Drug Delivery

4. New Potential and Characterization of Andrographis echioides L. Ness Stem Extract as an Anti-Arthritic Agent

5. Applications of Chitosan Microspheres as Drug Delivery Vehicles

The target audience comprises scholars and specialists in the field.

Brajesh Kumar
TATA College,
Kolhan University,
Chaibasa, India

Chapter 1

pH-Sensitive Carbonate Apatite Nanoparticles Facilitate the Delivery of siRNA in Breast Cancer Cells

Mohammad Borhan Uddin, Abdullah All Mamun Bhuiyan and Ratin Al Samir

Abstract

Recent advancements in nanotechnology have significantly enhanced the effectiveness of cancer treatments by enabling the precise targeting of tumour cells in the body. The integration of biological sciences and nanotechnology is poised to transform the field of cancer medicine in the coming century. Several therapeutic nanoparticles have already been approved for clinical use, with pH-sensitive carbonate apatite (CA) nanoparticles emerging as a promising option for cancer treatment. The use of pH-sensitive carbonate apatite nanoparticles as a delivery system for siRNA in cancer therapy has gained significant attention due to their ability to improve targeted delivery while minimizing off-target effects. Initially, these nanoparticles were utilized to encapsulate and deliver traditional chemotherapy drugs such as doxorubicin, cyclophosphamide, and gemcitabine *in vivo*, with the goal of reducing the side effects these drugs cause to healthy tissues. The fusion of biological sciences and nanotechnology is set to revolutionize cancer treatment in the coming years. Numerous therapeutic nanoparticles have already been authorized for clinical use, with pH-sensitive carbonate apatite nanoparticles (CA NPs) standing out as a promising candidate for cancer therapy. These nanoparticles were first explored for encapsulating and delivering conventional chemotherapy drugs like doxorubicin, cyclophosphamide, and gemcitabine *in vivo*, aiming to minimize the harmful side effects these drugs typically have on healthy tissues. Significant efforts have been made to enhance the productivity of CA particles, such as substituting the calcium component with strontium. These advancements have been highly successful, opening new possibilities for cancer treatment that move beyond traditional methods.

Keywords: carbonate apatite, nanoparticles, pH sensitivity, siRNA, breast cancer, gene therapy

1. Introduction

The most common type of cancer among women and the second biggest cause of deaths globally is breast cancer, making it one of the most difficult medical conditions to treat even in the twenty-first century [1]. Nowadays, adjuvant therapies such as hormonal, immunological, chemotherapy, or radiation therapies are routinely used in addition to surgery as part of cancer treatments. The lack of selectivity of these approaches is a major disadvantage, because medications such as cyclophosphamide, methotrexate, doxorubicin, cisplatin, 5-fluorouracil, and ionizing radiation have serious side effects in addition to killing cancer cells. One of the biggest problems with traditional cancer chemotherapy is still the toxicity of anticancer medications to healthy tissues [2]. The drug dosage must therefore be changed to a level that the body can handle without experiencing severe toxicity. Lowering the dosage, however, frequently makes the medication therapeutically ineffective, increasing the risk of cancer recurrence and chemoresistance [2]. The reduced uptake of drug molecules by target cancer cells and the emergence of drug resistance present additional difficulties for traditional cancer chemotherapy. The activity of multi-drug transporters that remove internalized medications from the cells and decrease therapeutic efficacy is frequently the cause of this resistance [2–4]. Efforts have been directed towards improving the distribution of medicines into cancer cells and prolonging the blood circulation period of both newly discovered and current medications. These methods seek to increase the effectiveness of killing cancer cells, reduce adverse effects, and pinpoint more exact treatment targets in different kinds of cancer cells [5, 6]. As a result, RNA interference has emerged as a promising strategy in the search for efficient cancer treatments. An essential RNAi technology, small-interfering RNA (siRNA), can be engineered to target silence genes that cause chemotherapeutic resistance and inactivity. Through the simultaneous suppression of target gene expression and improvement of chemotherapy efficacy, siRNA in combination with chemotherapeutic drugs provides a means of overcoming multidrug resistance (MDR). Furthermore, the synergistic or additive effects made possible by siRNA in combination therapy can greatly increase the therapeutic efficacy of chemotherapeutic medications. Particularly developed nanocarriers are necessary for the co-delivery of many chemotherapeutic agents. Although a variety of inorganic and organic nanomaterials smaller than a few hundred nanometers have lately surfaced as viable means of delivering siRNAs and chemotherapeutic drugs together, only few of these have shown promise. Carbonate apatite (CA) nanoparticles are especially well-suited for this use because of a number of their outstanding characteristics. These include good colloidal stability, beneficial pharmacokinetics, effective tumor absorption, strong ionic interactions with siRNAs and small molecule medicines, and intracellular disintegration in pH (acidic) of endosomes to release their therapeutic agent. These characteristics have helped siRNAs and chemotherapeutic medications be successfully delivered together in cell culture systems and animal models.

2. Nanotechnology in cancer therapy

Nanotechnology, which studies the structure, behavior, and properties of materials smaller than a few hundred nanometers, has advanced dramatically in recent years, producing nanoparticles with frequently modifiable characteristics [7–9], to eliminate the problems with the cancer treatment that is currently available [9], as well as uses in the additional fields of therapy. Ex. size variety of nanovehicle platforms between 10 and 200 nm that can be logically designed are ideal for high drug loading, preventing renal clearance and wide tissue distribution of small drugs, blocking nuclease-mediated siRNA by more precisely delivering the loaded drugs at the targeted site rather than at other healthy tissues, and artificially engineered nanoparticles could significantly increase the therapeutic efficiency of anticancer drugs while lowering non-specific toxicity, enabling safe and efficient cancer treatment [7]. To entirely achieve their effects, nanoparticles must be the right size, and 100 nm is typically thought to be the ideal size for passively targeting tumours *in vivo* [10]. Despite decades of research and development, only a small number of nanoparticle types have demonstrated encouraging therapeutic benefits when taking toxicity and efficacy into account [11], and pH-sensitive inorganic ions CA (Ca^{2+}, CO_3^{2-} and PO_4^{3-}) available in our body could be one of the potential candidates for clinical applications. After systemic administration, microRNA or doxorubicin is rapidly placed in tumour cells through endocytosis and rapidly dissolved in the pH (acidic) of endosomes, making it a pH-sensitive delivery mechanism. It should be emphasized that after being internalized into cells, drug-containing nanoparticles must quickly escape from increasingly acidic endosomes to prevent the pharmaceuticals from becoming further acidified and inactivated into lysosomes [4]. Therefore, CA's sensitivity to pH is very beneficial for releasing therapeutic cargo into the cytosol.

3. siRNAs in cancer therapy

Because of the overexpression or repression of different oncogenes, cancer is a disorder marked by aberrant and uncontrollable cell division that is frequently linked to malignant behaviours including invasion and metastasis [8]. Gene therapy is a collection of methods used to treat or prevent diseases by introducing exogenous DNA or RNA, either integrating or non-integrating, into living organisms to change gene expression. Since cancer is a genetic condition, gene therapy offers a promising treatment option. With more and more studies showing that RNAi is a promising gene alteration technology that may be employed either alone or in conjunction with other treatments, it has become a ground-breaking tool in gene therapy [7–9].

The development of cancer is often linked to the overexpression or suppression of certain signalling pathways that promote the growth and survival of cancer cells. One potential approach to make cancer cells more susceptible to chemotherapy is the targeted delivery of siRNAs, which can disrupt the gene transcripts of these pathways [12]. While traditional anticancer drugs trigger apoptosis in cancer cells by interfering with crucial cellular processes, including those involved in cell survival and proliferation, targeting specific genes that encode enzymes in these pathways could both reduce the proliferation of cancer cells and enhance their sensitivity to chemotherapy.

RNA interference is a technique for inhibiting the expression of particular genes or mRNA that may be used to create novel medications that target the desired therapeutic genes [6]. There are two ways to think about it: (1) nuclear delivery of gene expression cassettes that transcribe a short hairpin RNA, which is transformed into siRNA in the cytoplasm by further cellular machinery processing, and (2) cytoplasmic delivery of siRNA for consistently breaking down the target mRNA [8].

3.1 siRNA delivery challenges

A unique endogenous gene silencing mechanism known as RNA interference occurs when a small duplex RNA molecule degrades a specific mRNA. In recent years, it has been utilized extensively [11, 13], as a proper method for precisely regulating protein expression, particularly those that are typically thought to be nearly hard to target with traditional small molecule therapies. Previous studies have successfully used RNA interference as a technique to examine the consequences of knocking down certain genes. It has also been discovered that therapeutic administration of siRNA is effective in treating conditions like cancer [14].

However, because siRNA is unpleasant for distribution, its use as cancer therapies remains a major challenge. The first biological barrier to siRNA distribution is its vulnerability to nucleases, which quickly degrades it once it enters the body. This shortens its blood circulation period and restricts its therapeutic potential [11]. Delivering the siRNA to the right cells for its intended purposes is the next challenge. However, a weak connection between the siRNA and the cellular membrane occurs because of the negative charge of the oligonucleotides, which leads to low internalization into the target cells. As a result, siRNA delivery basically requires a vehicle [14]. Traditionally, physical techniques like electroporation and microinjection [15] were used to transfer siRNA into cells. However, these techniques are incompatible with the majority of *in vivo* applications. Allowing the internalized siRNA to leave the endosome in order to prevent its destruction and perform its biological roles in gene silencing is the final significant hurdle [11].

In order to get over these obstacles, siRNA has been added to a variety of formulations, such as virus-based delivery systems that use the short hairpin RNA (shRNA) sequence. While they work well for delivering shRNA-coding sequences to the nucleus, which then produces siRNA in cytosol [8], and due to the undesired gene mutation effects, the viral vector usage for the effective delivery has generated controversy [15].

For siRNA-based therapy to effectively deliver siRNA to the target area *in vivo*, a reliable and efficient carrier system is essential. One of the main challenges in gene therapy is developing a non-viral siRNA delivery system that is safe, effective, and capable of targeting specific cells. An ideal non-viral delivery system should ensure the release of siRNA in the correct intracellular compartment, have selectivity for specific tissues and cells, and protect the siRNA from degradation by serum proteins [7].

3.2 Ideal characteristics for siRNA delivery vehicles

The discovery of RNA interference in 1998 by Fire et al. [16], the first gene knockdown using siRNA in mammalian cells in 2001 [17], and the first clinical trial of siRNA for age-related macular degeneration in 2004 [18], sparked global interest in RNAi therapies. These therapies have shown great promise for treating a range of conditions, including cancer, liver diseases, and immune-related disorders. However, for the delivery vehicle to successfully transport siRNA and achieve its intended effects, it must meet several key requirements.

3.2.1 Bloodstream stability

The main objective of a siRNA delivery system is to maintain the stability of siRNA in the bloodstream after intravenous (IV) injection, as unprotected siRNA is quickly degraded by endogenous enzymes and aggregated by serum proteins. To prevent degradation or breakdown, the delivery system must be sufficiently stable and cohesive. Additionally, the carrier should have surface properties that facilitate interaction with the target cells while minimizing phagocytosis, immune activation, and nonspecific opsonization. Since naked siRNA is rapidly cleared from the blood within minutes of IV injection, prolonging its circulation time is also crucial for ensuring effective distribution [9].

3.2.2 Transport through the vascular endothelium

The endothelium increases the flow of materials into and out of tissues by acting as a semi-permeable barrier between the surrounding tissue and the vessel lumen. There are three forms of normal capillary endothelium: discontinuous capillaries, fenestrated capillaries, and continuous endothelium (**Figure 1**) [20]. In order to easily cross the weakly developed vasculature of solid tumors and inflammatory areas, where the increased permeability and retention (EPR) effect on drug delivery has been extensively documented, siRNA delivery methods should be tiny in size. In "leaky" tumor blood arteries, nanoparticles with less than 500 nm, often 150 nm or less diameter, demonstrated remarkable EPR effects [21].

3.2.3 The extracellular matrix's diffusion

For effective siRNA delivery, the carrier must first pass through the vascular endothelium and then diffuse into the extracellular matrix (ECM), which is composed of

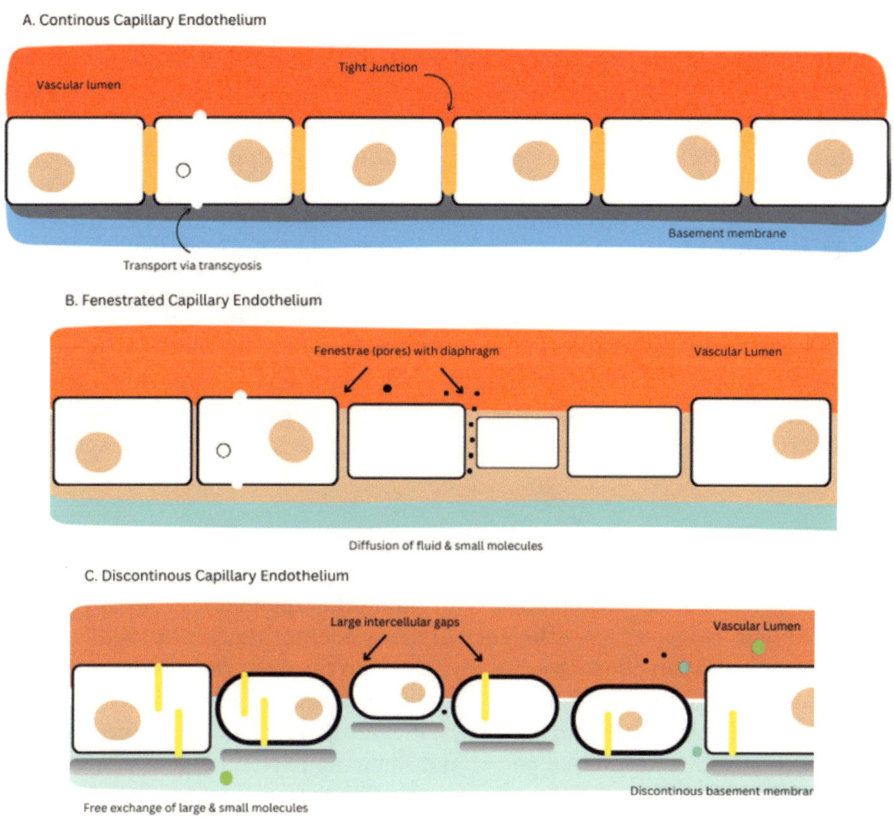

Figure 1.
Types of capillary endothelium [19].

fibrous proteins and polysaccharide gels that provide structural support to animal cells. In tumor tissue, where the ECM is tightly structured and has limited permeability, the diffusion of larger nanoparticles is hindered. Research by Cabral et al. demonstrated that nanoparticles smaller than 50 nm can penetrate tumor tissue effectively. For instance, 30-nm micelles were able to reach deep into pancreatic adenocarcinoma tissue, while 70-nm micelles were largely confined to the vasculature. Additionally, studies on human melanoma (Mu89) and glioblastoma (U87) showed that the diffusion of particles in the interstitial space decreases as their size increases. In U87 mouse tumors, the gap between aligned fibrils in the ECM was found to range from 20 to 42 nm, suggesting that smaller nanoparticles are more effective for delivering siRNA to tissues with limited permeability. Furthermore, research by Stylianopoulos et al. indicated that neutral particles diffuse faster than charged ones, highlighting the importance of nanoparticle charge in diffusion rates [22].

3.2.4 Transportation into the cytoplasm

Naked siRNA carries a negative charge. It is difficult to penetrate the cell membrane which is negatively charged. Therefore, siRNA is usually delivered using nanocarriers that are taken up by cells through endocytic pathways such as caveolae–/lipid raft-mediated endocytosis, clathrin-mediated endocytosis, or macropinocytosis [23, 24]. The delivery system of siRNA must first diffuse through the extracellular matrix, then cross the cell membrane and enter to the cytoplasm, and release the siRNA. The main mechanisms by which siRNA carriers are internalized into cells are clathrin-mediated endocytosis (CME) and macropinocytosis. These carriers are usually transported to endosomes once they are inside, where they finally combine with lysosomal vesicles. Because of the enzymatic breakdown caused by this association, endosomal escape techniques are required to guarantee efficient siRNA distribution. The caveolae–/lipid raft-mediated endocytosis pathway has received less research attention than macropinocytosis and CME [10]. Nevertheless, it has been shown that just a few of lipid raft-related delivery methods could directly carry medications into the cytosol without going *via* the endosomal pathway [25], opening the way for improved siRNA delivery in the cytosol. Different viral and nonviral siRNA delivery vehicles, such as lipid-based NPs, polymers or lipid polymer hybrid NPs, hydrogels, microbubbles, inorganic NPs, such as silica, gold, quantum dot, iron oxide, and carbon nanotubes, and other materials, such as oligonucleotide Nps and exosomes, have been created [26, 27] to overcome the obstacles related to the siRNA systemic transport.

3.3 Significance of siRNA in the cancer therapy

Cancer has historically been treated with chemotherapy medications as the first line of treatment. However, the efficiency of many chemotherapeutic medications that are typically used in clinics has decreased due to the drug resistance development and tumor heterogeneity [28]. Nucleic acid therapies and anticancer medications support chemotherapy in a number of ways, including by introducing apoptotic genes, restoring tumor suppressor genes, and silencing particular genes implicated in anti-apoptosis mechanisms and drug resistance. Either co-treatment with individual therapeutic drugs [29] or co-delivery of siRNA and anticancer drugs through a single carrier [30] can sum up chemotherapeutic drugs with siRNA; the latter is known to be more effective [31]. NPs carriers, which have the advantage of wrapping and releasing specific therapeutic compounds in a controlled manner at the appropriate spot, can be used to co-deliver several medicines [32]. Only a small number of nanoparticle carriers including polymer-based NPs, liposomes, and inorganic NPs have shown effective in co-delivering siRNA and chemotherapeutics. Because siRNA-based target gene silencing eventually boosts the cytotoxic drug activity, the co-delivery of chemotherapeutic drugs and siRNA *via* nanoparticles promotes the therapeutic response. Significant progress in siRNA-based cancer treatments has been made possible by the availability of many nanoparticle-based delivery technologies [33]. It has been discovered that delivery strategies based on nanoparticles increase the siRNA systemic stability, preventing premature degradation and facilitating quick *in vivo* clearance while fostering target-specific selectivity [11]. It has been discovered that employing siRNA in conjunction with other chemotherapeutic medications improves results by either increasing the cancer sensitivity to a therapeutic method or by acting in a synergistic or additive manner [34]. Since the development of nanoparticle carriers that support the integration of anticancer therapies, such as chemotherapeutic drugs, photodynamic sensitizers, or small molecule inhibitors, with siRNA, nano-drug delivery systems have increased the distribution of siRNA and other agents [35].

4. Delivery of siRNA in cancer therapy made better by inorganic CA nanoparticles

Viral and non-viral vehicles are used to transfer medicines based on nucleic acids. Despite the great gene transfer efficiency of viral delivery systems, their application has been restricted because of safety issues, mainly related to their immunogenic response. As a result, a lot of focus is now on developing non-viral vectors with better safety and effectiveness characteristics. Because of their remarkable performance in recent years, inorganic nanoparticles have drawn a lot of attention and been thoroughly researched for gene silencing applications among a variety of non-viral delivery mechanisms, including polymer-based nanoparticles, liposomes, and organic-inorganic hybrid materials.

Because of their remarkable physicochemical characteristics, inorganic nanoparticles make dependable vehicles for the co-delivery of siRNA and cancer drugs. These include stability in biological conditions, a wide surface area that is easily functionalized for medicinal compounds or ligands, a compact size, a high surface-area-to-volume ratio, and special optical or magnetic properties [36]. They are especially useful for designing RNA-based delivery systems for both *in vivo* and *in vitro* applications because of these characteristics [37, 38]. Through direct conjugation or non-covalent encapsulation, siRNA can be loaded efficiently into inorganic NPs due to their high surface area-to-volume ratio. One significant benefit of these NPs is that it is simple to alter their surface chemistry, which offers a way to get around the issues with siRNA distribution both *in vitro* and *in vivo* [20]. Moreover, siRNA transport to tissues or cells can be monitored using the unique optical and physical characteristics of inorganic NPs [39]. Physical characteristics such as size, elasticity, charge density, colloidal stability, and shape are crucial when developing nanoparticles since they dictate whether or not they are appropriate for a certain purpose [40]. Because of their distinct electrical and optical characteristics, ease of functionalization, biocompatibility, and minimal cytotoxicity, inorganic nanomaterials are currently in great demand [41]. Gold, silver, graphene oxide, calcium phosphate, quantum dots, and magnetic nanoparticles like iron oxides are a few examples of inorganic nanomaterials.

Inorganic carbonate apatite (CA) nanoparticles are formed through a chemical reaction involving Ca^{2+}, PO_4^{3-}, and HCO_3- resulting in a final crystal structure of $Ca_{10}(PO_4)_{6-X}(CO_3)_X(OH)_2$ with an diameter of 50–300 nm [4, 42, 43]. The size and number of CA particles produced depend on reaction such as calcium and bicarbonate concentrations, pH, and temperature [43]. CA particles deliver drug molecules through their anion- and cation-binding domains, which facilitate electrostatic interactions with drugs. Their nanoscale dimensions enhance cellular uptake of drug-loaded particles. The heterogeneous charge distribution of CA particles, combined with their ability to limit crystal growth for nanoscale formation, enables efficient endocytosis. Additionally, their rapid dissolution kinetics in acidic endosomal compartments allow for effective therapeutic release [42–51]. These characteristics have made CA nanocrystals a potentially useful instrument for the intracellular administration of different medications. The lower pH of endosomal vesicles aids in the dissolution of the particles after internalization through endocytosis, releasing the related medications into the cytoplasm for therapeutic action [42].

NPs of CA have been engineered to target particular locations, such as cancer cells or solid tumors. Depending on variables including particle diameter, surface properties, solubility, and stability, they can either be enclosed within or bonded to the nanoparticle surface, making them efficient carriers for medications and siRNA. Over the past few decades, pH-sensitive nanoparticle-based drug delivery systems have shown remarkable success in cancer treatments because of the substantial pH fluctuation across various tissues and organs. These systems have a strong affinity for both nucleic acid therapies and traditional medications. CA nanoparticles complexed with nucleic acids have been demonstrated to enable extremely effective gene delivery *in vitro*. This is explained by a number of noteworthy characteristics of CA nanoparticles, such as their potent affinity for binding DNA, biodegradability, and biocompatibility, which make them a potentially useful tool for therapeutic applications [49]. Research has also demonstrated that CA nanoparticles dissolve quickly at endosomal acidic pH, which causes the bound DNA to be released quickly for high protein expression levels in a variety of cell types [43]. After being absorbed, carbonate apatite nanoparticles can be quickly broken down in the acidic vesicles of cells due to their pH sensitivity and nanoscale size without showing any signs of toxicity. Their distinct characteristic has made them a viable substitute for conventional non-viral cancer delivery methods. In animal models of solid tumors, including breast cancer, these nanoparticles have so far been effectively used to deliver molecular therapies such as siRNA and transgenes as well as traditional anticancer medications such as methotrexate and doxorubicin.

siRNAs are delivered to specific cancer cells using CA nanoparticles. Effective siRNA integration into carriers, the stability of siRNA-carrier complexes, biocompatibility, targeted administration, biodistribution, and general functionality are some of the major issues that have prompted the creation of siRNA delivery systems. A key aspect is stability. While too much stability in nanocarriers can delay siRNA release, reducing therapeutic efficacy and raising systemic exposure to nanocarriers, which may result in toxicity, too little stability can cause premature siRNA release before reaching the targeted therapeutic site. Biodegradable nanoparticles with a regulated lifespan are ideal for overcoming these obstacles. These nanoparticles can minimize systemic adverse effects by stabilizing and protecting siRNA until it is transferred to the target site and guaranteeing prompt destruction once its therapeutic goal has been met.

5. CA nanoparticles enable the delivery of siRNA to suppress the expression of the ROS1 gene in malignant cells, thereby enhancing the cells sensitivity to anticancer treatments

pH-sensitive carbonate apatite nanoparticles (NPs) [52] enable combined delivery of drugs and nucleic acids *via* endocytosis, with rapid release in the acidic environment of endosomes. These nanoparticles have been successfully used in animal models, including breast cancer, to deliver both molecular therapies and traditional anticancer drugs. Co-delivering siRNA targeting ROS1 with paclitaxel in MCF-7 breast cancer cells showed synergistic effects, making cells more sensitive to treatment. Carbonate apatite-mediated delivery of ROS1 siRNA significantly reduced AKT1 phosphorylation in the PI3K pathway and enhanced doxorubicin sensitivity in 4 T1 murine mammary carcinoma cells. However, no increased sensitivity to cisplatin or paclitaxel was observed with ROS1 silencing in 4 T1 cells.

6. Carbonate apatite (CA) nanoparticles effectively delivered NF-κB siRNA to modulate the therapeutic effects of conventional anticancer drugs in human cervical cancer cells

Traditional chemotherapy drugs such as cisplatin, doxorubicin, and paclitaxel effectively treat breast cancer but often cause toxicity to healthy cells, leading to inadequate dosing, chemoresistance, and tumour recurrence. Carbonate apatite nanoparticles that are sensitive to pH have demonstrated efficacy in delivering siRNA to inhibit genes such as cyclin B1 and ABCG2/ABCB1, hence promoting death in cancer cells. Although there was no synergy with cisplatin or paclitaxel, CA-mediated NF-κB siRNA delivery in HeLa cells enhanced chemosensitivity to doxorubicin[141]. Significant increases in cell mortality were observed when HeLa cells were treated with apatite/siRNA complexes in combination with 0.2 μM cisplatin, doxorubicin, and paclitaxel. Nanoparticle-assisted intra-tumoral delivery of Bcl-2/IGF-1R siRNAs and the p53 gene effectively synergizes to suppress tumour growth in immunocompetent mice [19].

7. Development and intra-cellular delivery of siRNA/CA NPs for efficient cyclin B1 gene knockdown

Due to the rapid breakdown in acidic endosomes, which facilitates the release of medicines, and their capacity to inhibit crystal development for nanoscale particle formation, which improves endocytosis, carbonate apatite nanoparticles are an effective delivery mechanism [19]. More effective than lipofectamine at silencing gene expression, these pH-sensitive nanoparticles with a significant affinity for siRNAs facilitate efficient endocytosis and endosomal escape. Cyclin B1 siRNA delivered intracellularly dramatically suppresses the development of cancer cells and makes HeLa cells more sensitive to doxorubicin and cisplatin.

8. Carbonate apatite nanoparticles enabled siRNA delivery to overcome MDR in cancer treatment

The ATP-binding Cassette (ABC) transporter system plays a crucial role in multidrug resistance by actively expelling drugs from cancer cells. ABCB1 was the first cytotoxic drug efflux pump identified and removes drugs such as anthracyclines, vinca alkaloids, and taxanes, intracellular drug levels reduction below the threshold needed for cell death (**Figure 2**). In breast cancer, poor chemotherapy response is often linked to ABCB1 gene expression [54]. ABCG2, another ABC transporter, was later identified in multidrug-resistant breast cancer cells.

Efforts to overcome MDR by modulating ABC transporter activity have faced challenges. First-generation modulators failed due to toxicity, while second-generation ones caused undesirable pharmacokinetic interactions, leaving no clinically approved drug to reverse MDR. A promising alternative is to enhance chemosensitivity by selectively silencing ABC transporter genes to prevent their biosynthesis.

Among the 24 FDA-approved breast cancer drugs, doxorubicin, paclitaxel, and cisplatin are widely used from different drug families. Despite being used in combination therapies for better outcomes, their non-specific distribution and cancer cells' ability to acquire MDR through genetic and epigenetic changes diminish their effectiveness.

Small-interfering RNAs, short double-stranded RNA molecules (21–28 nucleotides), effectively degrade specific mRNAs, blocking the production of targeted proteins [53]. Recently, siRNAs have been used *in vitro* to counteract ABC transporter-mediated drug efflux by targeting ABCG2 and ABCB1 transporters (**Figure 3**). Combining siRNA-based gene therapy with chemotherapy has shown success in overcoming MDR by suppressing MDR-related genes, enhancing chemosensitivity, and improving treatment outcomes [53].

Carbonate apatite, a pH-sensitive nanocarrier, has been shown to be a successful method for delivering siRNA across cell membranes. When used with anticancer medications, it effectively inhibits the cyclin B1 gene, which causes cervical cancer cells to undergo apoptosis. Depending on the drug dosage, CA-facilitated siRNA delivery that targeted ABCB1 or ABCG2 in MCF-7 cells markedly enhanced chemosensitivity to paclitaxel, doxorubicin, and cisplatin. Additionally, co-delivery of siRNAs that targeted the transcripts of the ABCB1 and ABCG2 genes significantly increased chemosensitivity in MCF-7 cells, indicating the reversal of multidrug resistance mediated by the ABC transporter [53].

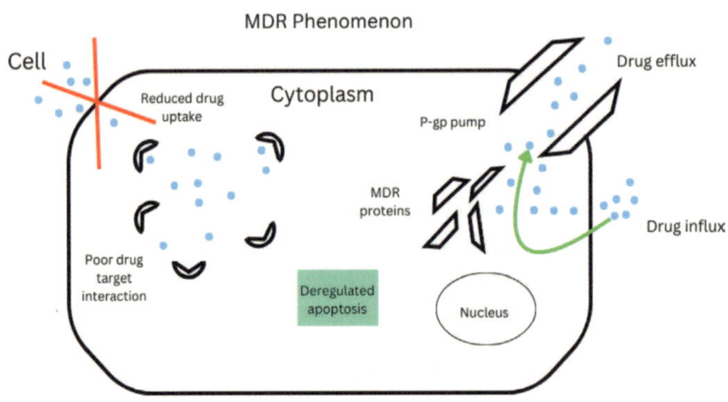

Figure 2.
MDR mechanisms in malignant cells [53].

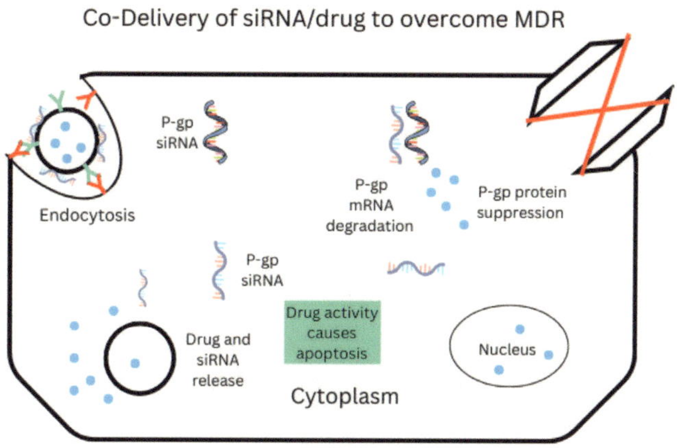

Figure 3.
Co delivery mechanism of siRNA and anticancer drug to overcome MDR [53].

9. CA NPs deliver siRNA targeting growth factor receptor genes, such as EGFR1 and ERBB2, effectively reducing breast tumor growth in mice

GFRs play a crucial role in cancer progression, and targeting these genes with siRNAs can reduce cancer cell aggressiveness by inhibiting growth and promoting cell death. In a study [55], it demonstrates that cells treated with CA NPs-bound negative control siRNA exhibited 80–90% viability, similar to NPs alone. However, siRNAs targeting EGFR1, ERBB2, and IGF1R resulted in 75.73%, 86.36%, and 78.11% viability, respectively. The siRNA targeting EGFR1 led to a significant decrease in cell viability ($p = 0.03$), while the siRNA targeting ERBB2 showed a trend towards reduced viability, though this was not statistically significant. No significant effect was observed with IGF1R-targeting siRNA [56].

10. Efficient breast cancer cell elimination *via* carbonate apatite nanoparticles mediating siRNA delivery to calcium ion channels

Western blot analysis was used to assess the activation of MAPK and AKT signalling pathways in MCF-7 cells treated with six CA-siRNA complexes, which showed strong cytotoxic effects. Both phosphorylated and unphosphorylated forms of MAPK and AKT were analysed, with GAPDH used for normalization. TRPC6 siRNA was combined with other siRNAs to explore potential synergistic effects on MAPK and AKT pathways, which are involved in calcium signalling and regulate cell proliferation and apoptosis. Treatment with siRNAs targeting TRPC6, TRPM8, and SLC41A1 showed reduced phospho-AKT levels and decreased total AKT expression, suggesting potential cross-talk between the AKT pathway and TRPC6. However, there was no significant change in MAPK activation. Other therapeutic targets, including TRPC6, TRPM7, and SLC41A1, showed promise for siRNA-mediated knockdown in breast cancer cells. The combined delivery of siRNAs targeting these calcium channels *via* carbonate apatite nanoparticles demonstrated a synergistic cytotoxic effect, indicating their potential for IV administration in breast cancer treatment [57].

11. Breast cancer inhibition *via* intravenous administration

of PRKCA siRNA- and PTEN tumour inhibitor gene by CA nanoparticlesAccording to Western blot and cell viability data [58], PRKCA has emerged as a possible target for siRNA-mediated knockdown, which could lower breast cancer cell survival and/or proliferation. Furthermore, gene augmentation treatment using CA NPs to deliver the PTEN tumor suppressor plasmid demonstrated a positive cell survival profile. Furthermore, by downregulating P-AKT, co-treatment of the plasmid and siRNA showed a remarkable decrease in breast cancer cell viability and a decreased level of proliferative signal.

12. A synergistic method for inhibiting the growth and survival of breast cancer cells: Hyaluronic acid-conjugated CA NPs for targeted delivery of siRNAs against ion channels and transporter genes

CD44 is a cell-surface multifunctional and multi-structural molecule, which plays a role in angiogenesis, cell proliferation, differentiation, and migration [59, 60]. Many cancer cells express CD44 at higher levels than normal cells, marking it an attractive target for cancer treatment.

Significant accumulations of basic CA nanoparticles were seen in the urinary system, RES organs (liver, spleen), and major organs (brain, heart), except for the lungs, which displayed stronger fluorescence signals. Hybrid hyaluronic acid (HA)-CA nanoparticles accumulated less in most organs. This might be because the hybrid particles are smaller, which speeds up renal clearance. By increasing their hydrodynamic diameter, the HA coating of CA NPs lessens accumulation in other organs. The EPR effect and the size of the tumours affect the accumulation of nanoparticles; more effective nanoparticle uptake is possible through tumour vascular holes. By interacting with CD44 receptors, hyaluronic acid may enhance siRNA-loaded targeting of hybrid carbonate apatite nanoparticles (CA NPs) to treat breast cancer. Since the nanoparticles dissolve rapidly in the acidic environment of the cell's endosomes following endocytosis, the biodegradable nature of the carrier aids in the effective release of the siRNAs. These findings imply that both pure and hybrid CA nanoparticles may be helpful in clinical settings for the delivery of therapeutic siRNAs, providing a viable strategy to target transporter genes and calcium ion channels to destroy breast cancer cells specifically [59].

13. Intracellular transport of siRNA *via* nano-carriers against integrin subunits to prevent the development of breast cancer cells

The use of CA-NPs to deliver integrin siRNAs led to a reduction in tumour volume compared to both untreated and CA-NP control groups. Significant tumour volume reductions ($p < 0.05$) were observed on days 11, 13, 15, 17, 19, 21, and 23 for the ITGαv + CA and ITGβ5 + CA treatments. The ITGα6 + CA treatment showed a significant decrease in tumour volume on days 11, 13, 15, 17, 19, and 21, while the ITGβ6 + CA treatment showed diminished tumour regression but still significant differences on days 17, 19, 21, and 23. **Table 1** details the tumour volume reduction compared to the CA-NP treated groups at various time points and demonstrates

Treatment	Day 10	Day 11	Day 13	Day 15	Day 17	Day 19	Day 21	Day 23
ITGαv + CA	2.12	2.32	2.12	1.99	2.10	1.68	1.70	1.71
ITGα6 + CA	2.43	2.40	1.68	2.44	2.65	2.42	2.05	1.5
ITGβ5 + CA	3.9	3.1	3.7	3.2	3.6	2.3	1.5	1.6
ITGβ6 + CA	1.8	2.51	1.5	1.6	1.7	1.7	1.7	1.7

Table 1.
Reduction of tumour in contrast to CA-NP treatment (Adapted with the permission of the author) [61].

Treatment	Day 10	Day 12	Day 14	Day 16	Day 19	Day 21	Day 23
ITGβ1 + CA	6.3	3.7	5.9	3.4	3.8	3.4	6.3
ITGβ + CA	3.84	4.90	4.11	3.50	4.87	3.54	3.69
ITGβ + CA	2.4	2.7	2.4	3.6	2.5	2.8	2.4

Table 2.
Reduction of tumour in comparison with CA-NP treatment (Adapted with the permission of the author) [61].

reduced tumour volumes using CA with ITGB1, ITGB2, ITGB3, and ITGB4 siRNA treatments. The untreated group was excluded from further experiments as no significant difference was observed between the untreated and CA-treated groups. Treatment with siRNA ITGβ1 + CA, ITGβ3 + CA, and ITGβ4 + CA resulted in a significant tumour size reduction ($p < 0.05$) at all time points compared to CA. **Table 2** shows the fold decrease in tumour volume relative to the CA control group on different days [61].

14. Delivery of siRNA intracellularly by aiming AKT and ERBB2 genes increases chemo-sensitization of breast cancer cells

Traditional breast cancer treatment includes drugs that are poorly absorbed and resistance has been developed against them. To improve this, the delivery of the drug along with siRNA targeting AKT and ERBB2 genes can give a successful result.

The human epidermal growth factor receptor (HER) family plays a key role in how breast cancer cells respond to chemotherapy. AKT, a protein kinase involved in cancer progression, is also critical. AKT activity is influenced by elevated HER signalling, RAS mutations that activate the PI3K pathway, or PTEN mutations that normally inhibit AKT. These alterations result in increased AKT activity, which can promote cancer progression and affect treatment effectiveness, even without an increase in AKT protein levels [62].

To assess the impact on ERBB2 protein expression levels, the effectiveness of various combinations of ERBB2 siRNA with paclitaxel or docetaxel was examined. The most significant knockdown was achieved when CA-bound docetaxel and ERBB2 siRNA were co-delivered, followed by the CA/paclitaxel/ERBB2 combination. These results clearly demonstrate a synergistic effect, with the combination of the drug and siRNA proving much more effective than using either the drug or siRNA alone [62, 63].

15. Challenges and future work recommendation

The use of pH-sensitive carbonate apatite nanoparticles for siRNA delivery in breast cancer cells presents several challenges that need to be overcome to optimize their therapeutic potential. One of the primary challenges is controlling the release of siRNA in the acidic environment of tumour cells. While CA is known to dissolve under acidic conditions, ensuring that the siRNA is released in a controlled and sustained manner is critical for achieving therapeutic efficacy. Additionally, the efficient cellular uptake of carbonate apatite nanoparticles is another hurdle, as the particles must be small enough to enter cells *via* endocytosis while being large enough to protect the siRNA from premature degradation. The surface charge and functionalization of the nanoparticles must be carefully optimized to improve cellular internalization and to avoid non-specific interactions with healthy tissues, which could lead to off target effects and toxicity. Biocompatibility is also a significant concern; while CA is generally considered biocompatible, long-term safety and potential cytotoxicity need thorough evaluation, especially when used for systemic delivery. Furthermore, ensuring specific targeting of cancer cells over normal cells remains challenging, as achieving precise localization and uptake at the tumour site is crucial for minimizing side effects and enhancing the therapeutic effect. Finally, scaling up the synthesis of CA nanoparticles in a cost-effective and reproducible manner for clinical applications remains a significant challenge [64].

Future work should focus on optimizing the surface properties of carbonate apatite nanoparticles, such as functionalizing them with targeting ligands (e.g., antibodies or peptides) to enhance their specificity for breast cancer cells. The specificity for the nanoparticles is a must cause they can damage normal cells by generating reactive oxygen species, inflammation, or by interrupting other cellular mechanisms. Personalized systems customized to various breast cancer subtypes need to be developed for better therapeutic activity and sophisticated stimuli-responsive delivery mechanisms should be introduced. Additionally, incorporating other biocompatible materials into the nanoparticle formulation could improve stability, facilitate endosomal escape, enhance the delivery of siRNA, and increase potency as CA nanoparticles can express its cytotoxicity at higher concentrations. Combining siRNA delivery with other therapies, such as chemotherapy or immunotherapy, could lead to synergistic effects, improving the overall therapeutic outcome. *In vivo* studies are necessary to assess the pharmacokinetics, biodistribution, and long-term safety of carbonate apatite nanoparticles, ensuring that they can be translated effectively from preclinical models to clinical applications. Furthermore, efforts to scale up production and standardize nanoparticle synthesis processes are essential to ensure consistent quality and reproducibility, which are critical for clinical trials and eventual commercialization. Addressing these challenges will help realize the full potential of pH-sensitive carbonate apatite nanoparticles as a promising delivery system for siRNA in breast cancer therapy [59, 65, 66].

16. Conclusion

In conclusion, pH-sensitive carbonate apatite nanoparticles (CA NPs) present a promising platform for the efficient delivery of siRNA in breast cancer therapy and siRNA therapeutics due to its unique optical and physical properties. Their ability to release siRNA selectively in the acidic tumour microenvironment enhances the targeted treatment of cancer cells while minimizing the risk of toxicity and other health issues. These include enhanced drug stability, endosomal escape, gene silencing, protection from rapid degradation, prolonged circulation, altered pharmacokinetics, and improved cellular uptake. CA nanoparticles leverage increased penetration and retention effects, allowing efficient targeting of tumour sites, higher therapeutic indices, and greater bioavailability compared to micron-sized particles. Their high surface area-to-volume ratio enables effective drug loading, and pH sensitivity ensures targeted delivery [67–69].

Furthermore, the biocompatibility and versatility of CA NPs open new avenues for combination therapies, where siRNA can be co-delivered with traditional chemotherapeutic agents. siRNA and anticancer drug's co-delivery using CA nanoparticles enhances therapeutic outcomes by achieving synergistic effects and overcoming multidrug resistance (MDR) through mechanisms like diverting drug efflux pumps. This approach allows simultaneous targeting of multiple pathways involved in cancer progression and resistance. Despite recent advancements, challenges like system complexity and the need to validate the safety of individual components remain. As research progresses, CA NPs have the potential to significantly advance the field of personalized cancer treatment, offering a novel and effective strategy for overcoming the limitations of current therapies in breast cancer.

Acknowledgements

The authors sincerely acknowledge the support provided by Professor Dr. Ezharul Hoque Chowdhury; Nanoflex LLC, Leesburg, FL, 34748, USA; Email: chowdhury@nanoflex-usa.com.

Funding

This particular research did not receive any funding from any government or non-government organizations.

Conflict of interest

There is no conflict of interest.

Author details

Mohammad Borhan Uddin*, Abdullah All Mamun Bhuiyan and Ratin Al Samir
Department of Pharmaceutical Sciences, School of Health and Life Sciences, North South University, Dhaka, Bangladesh

*Address all correspondence to: mohammad.uddin@northsouth.edu
and bnn.nsu@gmail.com

References

[1] Peer D, Karp JM, Hong S, Farokhzad OC, Margalit R, Langer R. Nanocarriers as an emerging platform for cancer therapy. 1st ed. Nano-enabled Medical Applications; Nov 2020. pp. 61-91

[2] Hossain S, Yamamoto H, Chowdhury EH, Wu X, Hirose H, Haque A, et al. Fabrication and intracellular delivery of doxorubicin/carbonate apatite nanocomposites: Effect on growth retardation of established colon tumor. PLoS One. 2013;**8**(4):e60428

[3] Varkouhi AK, Scholte M, Storm G, Haisma HJ. Endosomal escape pathways for delivery of biologicals. Journal of Controlled Release. 2011;**151**(3):220-228

[4] Chowdhury EH, Kunou M, Nagaoka M, Kundu AK, Hoshiba T, Akaike T. High-efficiency gene delivery for expression in mammalian cells by nanoprecipitates of Ca–Mg phosphate. Gene. 2004;**341**:77-82

[5] Chowdhury EH. Strategies for tumor-directed delivery of siRNA. Expert Opinion on Drug Delivery. 2011;**8**(3):389-401

[6] Burnett JC, Rossi JJ. RNA-based therapeutics: Current progress and future prospects. Chemistry & Biology. 2012;**19**(1):60-71

[7] Thomas CE, Ehrhardt A, Kay MA. Progress and problems with the use of viral vectors for gene therapy. Nature Reviews Genetics. 2003;**4**(5):346-358

[8] Vorhies JS, Nemunaitis J. Nonviral delivery vehicles for use in short hairpin RNA-based cancer therapies. Expert Review of Anticancer Therapy. 2007;7(3):373-382

[9] Alexis F, Pridgen E, Molnar LK, Farokhzad OC. Factors affecting the clearance and biodistribution of polymeric nanoparticles. Molecular Pharmaceutics. 2008;**5**(4):505-515

[10] Bareford LM, Swaan PW. Endocytic mechanisms for targeted drug delivery. Advanced Drug Delivery Reviews. 2007;**59**(8):748-758

[11] Whitehead KA, Langer R, Anderson DG. Knocking down barriers: Advances in siRNA delivery. Nature Reviews Drug Discovery. 2009;**8**(2):129-138

[12] Jiang S, Eltoukhy AA, Love KT, Langer R, Anderson DG. Lipidoid-coated iron oxide nanoparticles for efficient DNA and siRNA delivery. Nano Letters. 2013;**13**(3):1059-1064

[13] Aagaard L, Rossi JJ. RNAi therapeutics: Principles, prospects and challenges. Advanced Drug Delivery Reviews. 2007;**59**(2-3):75-86

[14] Schiffelers RM, Ansari A, Xu J, Zhou Q, Tang Q, Storm G, et al. Cancer siRNA therapy by tumor selective delivery with ligand-targeted sterically stabilized nanoparticle. Nucleic Acids Research. 2004;**32**(19):e149

[15] Hiruta C, Toyota K, Miyakawa H, Ogino Y, Miyagawa S, Tatarazako N, et al. Development of a microinjection system for RNA interference in the water flea *Daphnia pulex*. BMC Biotechnology. 2013;**13**:1-7

[16] Fire A, Xu S, Montgomery MK, Kostas SA, Driver SE, Mello CC. Potent and specific genetic interference by double-stranded RNA in *Caenorhabditis elegans*. Nature. 1998;**391**(6669):806-811

[17] Elbashir SM, Harborth J, Lendeckel W, Yalcin A, Weber K, Tuschl T. Duplexes of 21-nucleotide RNAs mediate RNA interference in cultured mammalian cells. Nature. 2001;**411**(6836):494-498

[18] Whelan J. First clinical data on RNAi. Drug Discovery Today. 2005;**10**(15):1014-1015

[19] Stanislaus A, Hossain S, Chua MJ, Kunnath AP, Wen QC, Syakira SN, et al. Fabrication and intracellular delivery of siRNA/carbonate apatite nano-composites for effective knockdown of cyclin B1 gene. Drugs and Therapy Studies. 2011;**1**(1):e8. DOI: 10.4081/dts.2011.e8

[20] Takakura Y, Mahato RI, Hashida M. Extravasation of macromolecules. Advanced Drug Delivery Reviews. 1998;**34**(1):93-108

[21] Li W, Szoka FC. Lipid-based nanoparticles for nucleic acid delivery. Pharmaceutical Research. 2007;**24**:438-449

[22] Cabral H, Matsumoto Y, Mizuno K, Chen Q, Murakami M, Kimura M, et al. Accumulation of sub-100 nm polymeric micelles in poorly permeable tumours depends on size. Nature Nanotechnology. 2011;**6**(12):815-823

[23] Petros RA, DeSimone JM. Strategies in the design of nanoparticles for therapeutic applications. Nature Reviews Drug Discovery. 2010;**9**(8):615-627

[24] Conner SD, Schmid SL. Regulated portals of entry into the cell. Nature. 2003;**422**(6927):37-44

[25] Partlow KC, Lanza GM, Wickline SA. Exploiting lipid raft transport with membrane targeted nanoparticles: A strategy for cytosolic drug delivery. Biomaterials. 2008;**29**(23):3367-3375

[26] Semple SC, Akinc A, Chen J, Sandhu AP, Mui BL, Cho CK, et al. Rational design of cationic lipids for siRNA delivery. Nature Biotechnology. 2010;**28**(2):172-176

[27] Truong NP, Gu W, Prasadam I, Jia Z, Crawford R, Xiao Y, et al. An influenza virus-inspired polymer system for the timed release of siRNA. Nature Communications. 2013;**4**(1):1902

[28] Dexter DL, Leith JT. Tumor heterogeneity and drug resistance. Journal of Clinical Oncology. 1986;**4**(2):244-257

[29] Tekedereli I, Alpay SN, Akar U, Yuca E, Ayugo-Rodriguez C, Han HD, et al. Therapeutic silencing of Bcl-2 by systemically administered siRNA nanotherapeutics inhibits tumor growth by autophagy and apoptosis and enhances the efficacy of chemotherapy in orthotopic xenograft models of ER (−) and ER (+) breast cancer. Molecular Therapy-Nucleic Acids. 2013;**2**:e121

[30] Shen Y, Wang J, Li Y, Tian Y, Sun H, Ammar O, et al. Co-delivery of siRNA and paclitaxel into cancer cells by hyaluronic acid modified redox-sensitive disulfide-crosslinked PLGA–PEI nanoparticles. RSC Advances. 2015;**5**(58):46464-46479

[31] Creixell M, Peppas NA. Co-delivery of siRNA and therapeutic agents using nanocarriers to overcome cancer resistance. Nano Today. 2012;**7**(4):367-379

[32] Godsey ME, Suryaprakash S, Leong KW. Materials innovation for co-delivery of diverse therapeutic cargos. RSC Advances. 2013;**3**(47):24794-24811

[33] Yin H, Kanasty RL, Eltoukhy AA, Vegas AJ, Dorkin JR, Anderson DG. Non-viral vectors for gene-based

therapy. Nature Reviews Genetics. 2014;**15**(8):541-555

[34] Xiao B, Ma L, Merlin D. Nanoparticle-mediated co-delivery of chemotherapeutic agent and siRNA for combination cancer therapy. Expert Opinion on Drug Delivery. 2017;**14**(1):65-73

[35] Saraswathy M, Gong S. Recent developments in the co-delivery of siRNA and small molecule anticancer drugs for cancer treatment. Materials Today. 2014;**17**(6):298-306

[36] Jiang Y, Huo S, Hardie J, Liang XJ, Rotello VM. Progress and perspective of inorganic nanoparticle-based siRNA delivery systems. Expert Opinion on Drug Delivery. 2016;**13**(4):547-559

[37] Zhang L, Li Y, Jimmy CY. Chemical modification of inorganic nanostructures for targeted and controlled drug delivery in cancer treatment. Journal of Materials Chemistry B. 2014;**2**(5):452-470

[38] Zhao MX, Zeng EZ, Zhu BJ. The biological applications of inorganic nanoparticle drug carriers. ChemNanoMat. 2015;**1**(2):82-91

[39] Lim EK, Kim T, Paik S, Haam S, Huh YM, Lee K. Nanomaterials for theranostics: Recent advances and future challenges. Chemical Reviews. 2015;**115**(1):327-394

[40] Sattler KD. Handbook of Nanophysics: Nanomedicine and Nanorobotics. USA: CRC Press; 2010

[41] Erathodiyil N, Ying JY. Functionalization of inorganic nanoparticles for bioimaging applications. Accounts of Chemical Research. 2011;**44**(10):925-935

[42] Chowdhury EH, Maruyama A, Kano A, Nagaoka M, Kotaka M, Hirose S, et al. pH-sensing nano-crystals of carbonate apatite: Effects on intracellular delivery and release of DNA for efficient expression into mammalian cells. Gene. 2006;**376**(1):87-94

[43] Chowdhury EH, Akaike T. High performance DNA nano-carriers of carbonate apatite: Multiple factors in regulation of particle synthesis and transfection efficiency. International Journal of Nanomedicine. 2007;**2**(1):101-106

[44] Hossain S, Stanislaus A, Chua MJ, Tada S, Tagawa YI, Chowdhury EH, et al. Carbonate apatite-facilitated intracellularly delivered siRNA for efficient knockdown of functional genes. Journal of Controlled Release. 2010;**147**(1):101-108

[45] Hossain S, Tada S, Akaike T, Chowdhury EH. Influences of electrolytes and glucose on formulation of carbonate apatite nanocrystals for efficient gene delivery to mammalian cells. Analytical Biochemistry. 2010;**397**(2):156-161

[46] Hossain S, Chowdhury EH, Akaike T. Nanoparticles and toxicity in therapeutic delivery: The ongoing debate. Therapeutic Delivery. 2011;**2**(2):125-132

[47] Tada S, Chowdhury EH, Cho CS, Akaike T. pH-sensitive carbonate apatite as an intracellular protein transporter. Biomaterials. 2010;**31**(6):1453-1459

[48] Kutsuzawa K, Akaike T, Chowdhury EH. The influence of the cell-adhesive proteins E-cadherin and fibronectin embedded in carbonate-apatite DNA carrier on transgene delivery and expression in a mouse embryonic stem cell line. Biomaterials. 2008;**29**(3):370-376

[49] Chowdhury EH. pH-sensitive nano-crystals of carbonate apatite for smart

and cell-specific transgene delivery. Expert Opinion on Drug Delivery. 2007;**4**(3):193-196

[50] Chowdhury EH, Akaike T. Bio-functional inorganic materials: An attractive branch of gene-based nano-medicine delivery for 21st century. Current Gene Therapy. 2005;**5**(6):669-676

[51] Chowdhury EH, Akaike T. A bio-recognition device developed onto nano-crystals of carbonate apatite for cell-targeted gene delivery. Biotechnology and Bioengineering. 2005;**90**(4):414-421

[52] Tiash S, Chua MJ, Chowdhury EH. Knockdown of ROS1 gene sensitizes breast tumor growth to doxorubicin in a syngeneic mouse model. International Journal of Oncology. 2016;**48**(6):2359-2366

[53] Babu A, Munshi A, Ramesh R. Combinatorial therapeutic approaches with RNAi and anticancer drugs using Nanodrug delivery systems. Drug Development and Industrial Pharmacy. 2017;**43**(9):1391-1401

[54] Tiwari AK, Sodani K, Chen ZS. Current advances in modulation of ABC transporter-mediated multidrug resistance in cancer. International Journal of Toxicological and Pharmacological Research. 2009;**1**:1-6

[55] Tiash S, Kamaruzman NI, Chowdhury EH. Carbonate apatite nanoparticles carry siRNA (s) targeting growth factor receptor genes egfr1 and erbb2 to regress mouse breast tumor. Drug Delivery. 2017;**24**(1):1721-1730

[56] Knowlden JM, Hutcheson IR, Jones HE, et al. Elevated levels of epidermal growth factor receptor/c-erbB2 heterodimers mediate an autocrine growth regulatory pathway in tamoxifen-resistant MCF-7 cells. Endocrinology. 2003;**144**:1032-1044

[57] Uddin MB, Balaravi Pillai B, Tha KK, Ashaie M, Karim ME, Chowdhury EH. Carbonate apatite nanoparticles-facilitated intracellular delivery of siRNA(s) targeting calcium ion channels efficiently kills breast cancer cells. Toxics. 2018;**6**(3):34. DOI: 10.3390/toxics6030034

[58] Ibnat N, Islam RA, Chowdhury EH. Inhibition of breast tumour growth with intravenously administered PRKCA siRNA-and PTEN tumour suppressor gene-loaded carbonate apatite nanoparticles. Applied Sciences. 2021;**11**(17):8133

[59] Uddin MB, Holl MMB, Chowdhury EH. Delivery of siRNAs against selective ion channels and transporter genes using hyaluronic acid-coupled carbonate apatite nanoparticles synergistically inhibits growth and survival of breast cancer cells. International Journal of Nanomedicine. 2024;**19**:7709-7727. DOI: 10.2147/IJN.S440419

[60] Lau WM, Teng E, Chong HS, et al. CD44v8-10 is a cancer-specific marker for gastric cancer stem cells. Cancer Research. 2014;**74**(9):2630-2641. DOI: 10.1158/0008-5472.CAN-13-2309

[61] Ashaie M, Chowdhury EH. Nanoparticles-facilitated intracellular transport of siRNAs against individual integrin subunits inhibits growth of breast cancer cells. Applied Sciences. 2021;**11**(22):10782

[62] Fatemian T, Moghimi HR, Chowdhury EH. Intracellular delivery of siRNAs targeting AKT and ERBB2 genes enhances chemosensitization of breast cancer cells in a culture and animal model. Pharmaceutics. 2019;**11**(9):458

[63] Chua MJ, Tiash S, Fatemian T, et al. Carbonate apatite-facilitated intracellular delivery of c-ROS1 small interfering RNA sensitises MCF-7 breast cancer cells to cisplatin and paclitaxel. OA Cancer. 2013;**1**:1-9

[64] Ghosh S, Dutta S, Sarkar A, Kundu M, Sil PC. Targeted delivery of curcumin in breast cancer cells via hyaluronic acid modified mesoporous silica nanoparticle to enhance anticancer efficiency. Colloids and Surfaces, B: Biointerfaces. 2021;**197**:111404. DOI: 10.1016/j.colsurfb.2020.111404

[65] Hossain SM, Zainal Abidin SA, Chowdhury EH. Krebs cycle intermediate-modified carbonate apatite nanoparticles drastically reduce mouse tumor burden and toxicity by restricting broad tissue distribution of anticancer drugs. Cancers. 2020;**12**(1):161. DOI: 10.3390/cancers12010161

[66] Karim ME, Shetty J, Islam RA, Kaiser A, Bakhtiar A, Chowdhury EH. Strontium sulfite: A new pH-responsive inorganic nanocarrier to deliver therapeutic siRNAs to cancer cells. Pharmaceutics. 2019;**11**(2):89. DOI: 10.3390/pharmaceutics11020089

[67] Karim ME, Tha KK, Othman I, Borhan Uddin M, Chowdhury EH. Therapeutic potency of nanoformulations of siRNAs and shRNAs in animal models of cancers. Pharmaceutics. 2018;**10**(2):65. DOI: 10.3390/pharmaceutics10020065

[68] Chowdhury EH. Nanotherapeutics: From Laboratory to Clinic. USA: CRC Press; 2016

[69] Ibnat N, Zaman R, Uddin MB, Chowdhury E, Lee CY. Improved systemic half-life of glucagon-like peptide-1-loaded carbonate apatite nanoparticles in rats. World Journal of Diabetes. 2022;**13**(8):613

Chapter 2

Albumin as a Drug Delivery System: Mechanisms, Applications, and Innovations

Samah Al-Harthi, Awatef Alshehri, Lubna Alhudhali, Mawadda Alghrably, Giulia Bennici, Maram Almohaywi, Łukasz Jaremko and Mariusz Jaremko

Abstract

Albumin, the most abundant plasma protein, has emerged as a promising carrier in drug delivery because of its exceptional biocompatibility, stability, and ligand-binding capacity. This chapter explored the role of albumin-based drug delivery systems and focused on their mechanism, recent innovations, and applications. Albumin can bind endogenous and exogenous molecular facilities for transport and controlled release of therapeutic agents, improve drug bioavailability, and minimize adverse effects. It has a long circulatory half-life facilitated by the neonatal Fc receptor (FcRn). This ensures a prolonged, systematic exposure, which makes it a viable option for targeted and sustained drug release. A chapter delves into a multiple drug-binding mechanism, including covalent and noncovalent interactions, nanoparticle formulation, and nanoparticles. The albumin nanoparticles (ABNPs) are particularly significant in modern therapeutics, controlled drug release, enhanced solubility, and tumor targets through receptor-mediated uptake and enhanced permeability and retention (EPR) effects. Through preparation techniques, like desolvation, emulsification, and high-pressure homogenization (NAB™ technology), they optimized an albumin nanoparticle for the enhancement of therapeutic efficacy. A clinical application of the albumin-based system extended beyond oncology, with notable success in diabetes, neurodegenerative disorders, and infectious diseases. The engineered albumin variant and albumin-drug conjugates expand the versatility of precision medicine. Challenges like stability, manufacturing scalability, and the drug-albumin interactions required continued refinement of albumin's role in drug delivery.

Keywords: albumin-based drug delivery, nanocarriers, therapeutic applications, ligand binding, targeted drug delivery

1. Introduction

Albumin is the most abundant plasma protein and has been extensively studied. Its presence is crucial for clinical monitoring, physiology, and therapy. It is produced in the liver and then present in the circulatory system. This consists of approximately 60% of the total protein content in the human body [1–4]. About 80% of the plasma oncotic pressure is supplied by it, guaranteeing an adequate fluid distribution between tissues and blood vessels. This is produced at 10.5 g/day, with a turnover time of around 25 days. This is eliminated by the kidneys (about 6%), the gastrointestinal tract (approximately 10%), and this cationization process (approximately 84%) [5]. The human serum albumin (HSA) gene encoded a pre-ovalbumin, a 609 amino acid translation product with a molecular mass of 69.3 kDa [1]. Albumin is produced in the liver and undergoes posttranslational modification in the Golgi apparatus. The first 24 amino acids are cleaved before being released into the bloodstream.

Albumin is essential to preserving physiological homeostasis because it plays a role in molecular binding and colloidal osmotic pressure [3]. There are several types of albumin, like Bovine Serum Albumin (BSA), human serum albumin (HSA), rat serum albumin (RSA), and egg white (OVA), and OVA is frequently utilized as a food source in research [6]. The BSA is commonly employed in laboratory settings for various biochemical purposes. The RSA has been used in animal studies to study human albumin activities [3]. The BSA is frequently employed in laboratory settings for various biochemical issues, and there are some notable similarities in sequence, structure, and surface charge distribution between HSA and BSA [1]. The HSA and BSA have 76% sequence-level identity, and serum albumin from different sources shared more than 62% overall.

The structure of a mature HSA is a monomeric, globular, mostly α-helical protein composed of 585 amino acids. This forms a heart-shaped protein comprised of three topologically identical and structure-related domains (I, II, and III), each subdivided into subdomains (A and B). This is only a free cysteine (Cys34), supported by 17 disulfide bridges. This has several binding sites: Sudlow's Site I and II (for drugs), the presence of nine fatty acid binding sites, as well as four metal-binding sites [1, 4, 7, 8]. Furthermore, on the binding sites, the N-terminal sequence (Asp1–Ala2–His3) binds a transition metal like Cu^{2+} and Ni^{2+}, while a primary metal-binding site (MBS-A) at a domain I/II interface binds Zn^{2+} and Cd^{2+} [9]. At the same time, the N-terminal sequence (Asp1–Ala2–His3) binds a transition metal just like Cu^{2+}, Ni^{2+}, and Cd^{2+} [9]. For a thorough review of an albumin's structural characteristics and its dynamics, refer to [1].

The conformational flexibility of HSA, manipulated by the ligands, specifically when fatty acids are bound, affects its ability to bind metals and drugs. HSA's ability to interact with many biological molecules depends on the presence of both positive and negative charge regions on a surface [10]. In addition, albumin serves as the carrier protein, binding transportation by a range of substances to regulate its metabolism and bioavailability. This includes hormones, fatty acids, zinc, calcium, and pharmaceuticals [1, 2]. The HSA has been used therapeutically since the 1940s, and this is the first treatment to burn a patient at Pearl Harbor in the year 1941. This shows that HSA may be used to treat cirrhosis [11]. A therapeutic application that has been extended to a variety of clinical contexts, such as hypovolemia and hypoalbuminemia [12]. HSA holds significant promise in various novel therapeutic areas in addition to its traditional use [2, 3, 6]. One promising method is drug delivery to generate albumin-based nanoparticles (NPs). These NPs can bind a wider range of molecules and have greater features like nontoxicity, biodegradability, and biocompatibility. NPs are a great carrier for various advanced therapeutics, including small molecules, proteins, and peptides [13]. There are a few methods for generating albumin NPs, such as self-assembly, nab technology, thermal gelation, desolvation, emulsification, and no spray drying [6].

DOI: http://dx.doi.org/10.5772/intechopen.1011323

2. Properties of albumin favorable for drug delivery

For the drug to have a high therapeutic efficacy, it needs to be available at the target site of action at a certain rate and concentration, which can enhance the effectiveness and reduce patient adverse effects [4, 14–16]. Nonetheless, challenges associated with the drug's nonspecific accumulation, renal clearance, and degradation require the exploration of innovative and alternative drug delivery systems to tackle these issues. Among the promising drug carriers, albumin is distinguished as an exceptional macromolecular vehicle, demonstrating features that render it a compelling option for drug delivery in clinical and industrial applications [3, 17]. Albumin is a highly abundant and water-soluble protein involved in naturally transporting a wide range of molecules because of its extraordinary binding capacity facilitated by multiple ligand-binding sites [18, 19]. Hence, albumin is a pivotal contender as a molecular cargo for drug delivery owing to its high solubility, stability, nontoxicity, biodegradability, natural ligand-binding capacity, long circulatory half-life, biocompatibility, and nonimmunogenicity [4]. These characteristics render albumin an essential carrier for drug transport, facilitating improved pharmacokinetics, targeted delivery, and enhanced drug stability [3, 16, 20, 21]. Leveraging the features of albumin positions it as an excellent contender for advancing next-generation drug delivery systems.

2.1 High solubility and stability

Albumin, a crucial plasma protein, demonstrates maximum solubility in aqueous solutions at neutral pH due to its surface's prevalence of charged amino acids [15]. Albumin comprises 98 acidic amino acids (glutamic acid and aspartic acid) and 83 basic amino acids (lysine and arginine) on its surface, which is gaining interest as a potential delivery mechanism for sugars, peptides, and poorly water-soluble drugs [22]. Moreover, its high solubility facilitates delivery *via* injection, rendering it a suitable candidate for nanoparticle formulation. Albumin demonstrates substantial stability against variations in pH, thermal conditions, and denaturing solvents [15]. The molecule comprises 35 cysteine residues, with 34 involved in establishing internal disulfide bridges in its structure, significantly enhancing the albumin's stability [22]. It demonstrates stability across a wide pH range of 4–9 and is soluble in 40% ethanol [20]. It exhibits minimal stability at elevated temperatures, enduring heating at 60°C for up to 10 hours without negative consequences. The characteristics of carriers, such as albumin, are essential for maintaining structural integrity under physiological conditions, thus preserving the encapsulated or bound therapeutic agents from premature degradation during transport and storage. These characteristics facilitate the development of long-acting injectable formulations. Albumin-bound formulations, such as nab-paclitaxel, leverage stability properties to enhance drug solubility efficacy, extend drug release duration, and decrease dosing frequency.

2.2 Natural ligand-binding capacity

Albumin (BSA and HSA) has a remarkable ability to bind to various molecules, making it an attractive nanoparticle carrier system [7, 16, 23]. It can bind to a wide range of endogenous and exogenous molecules, including fatty acids (i.e., myristate), drugs (i.e., ibuprofen or warfarin), hormones (i.e., thyroxine), and metal ions [1]. These compounds can be embedded into the albumin matrix due to the presence of several binding sites for organic and inorganic molecules across its three domains.

Depending on the location of the site, different types of molecules can interact, including ions, water-repelling (hydrophobic) or water-attracting (hydrophilic) molecules, and the location of the site [24]. This binding capacity not only aids in transporting essential compounds, drugs, and waste materials within the circulatory system, but it also improves the absorption of hydrophobic drugs and neutralizes circulating toxins until the liver or kidneys can eliminate them. Importantly, albumin serves as a depot, facilitating the gradual release of drugs over time, which enhances available quantities, improves pharmacokinetics, and reduces dosing frequency [6].

BSA and HSA show distinct affinities for similar ligands, owed to variations in their amino acid composition that influence the structure and characteristics of their ligand-binding sites. They have about 76% similarity in their sequence; however, differences in crucial residues result in variations in their hydrophobic properties, charge distribution, and ability to form hydrogen bonds, which impact their binding capabilities [7, 25]. These differences ultimately determine the specificity of their interactions with ligands. Ligand binding occurs in Sudlow sites (I and II) and other hydrophobic pockets, where variations in residue composition, structural flexibility, and tertiary interactions lead to various binding characteristics [26]. For example, substituting polar or charged amino acids with nonpolar residues can modify the binding affinities, affecting ligand binding. The isoelectric point (pl) of the HSA is roughly 4.7, which is slightly acidic compared to BSA, which leads to a pl. of around 5.4 [6]. A difference affects its interaction with charged ligands. Furthermore, post-translational modifications such as glycosylation and oxidation, which are more common in HSA than BSA, can further influence binding [24, 27]. The variation in hydrophobic surface areas contributed significantly, as HSA generally exhibits greater efficiency in binding fatty acid drugs because of appropriate structured hydrophobic regions [1, 4, 23]. HSA has demonstrated a higher affinity for warfarin, which is attributed to the presence of Trp 24 in a Sudlow Site. At the same time, the BSA's absence of residue diminishes efficiency [28]. It is essential to recognize species variations to understand how albumin functions in drug delivery systems, particularly in improving its efficiency in transporting and binding substances for therapeutic use [29].

2.3 Long circulatory half-life

On average, an albumin-extended blood circulatory half-life is 9–21 days in vivo [4]. In vivo, the characteristics make it a viable carrier for drug delivery, and this enables the transportation of hydrophobic drugs across different barriers and extends drug retention [3, 16, 17]. A prolonged half-life is regulated by a megalin/cubilin-complex rescue from the renal clearance, and this is, most importantly, by a broadly expressed cellular receptor called a neonatal Fc receptor [3, 27, 30]. This receptor-mediated recycling helps the albumin evade intracellular degradation. It facilitates protein recycling to the bloodstream through a strictly pH-dependent recycling mechanism where albumin binds to the receptor with high-affinity binding at low pH in the acid endosome and diverts them from a lysosomal pathway, then it returns to the extracellular compartment, where it is released at physiological pH, thus extending their half-lives [3]. Therefore, FcRn is essential for the homeostatic regulation of albumin, ensuring extensive biological distribution throughout the body. This feature ensures prolonged drug delivery and enhanced therapeutic effectiveness as a drug carrier. For example, albumin-based nanoparticles employ this technique to prolong the circulation of therapeutic drugs, hence increasing drug accumulation at target areas and reducing off-target effects [21].

Additionally, the chemical coupling of polyethylene glycol (PEG) to a protein, referred to as PEGylation, is a potential way to improve nanoparticles' blood circulatory half-life by more than 50-fold. Albumin-based nanoparticles present numerous possibilities for surface modification, attributed to functional groups such as carboxylic and amino groups on their surface [31]. This study by Fahrländer et al. confirmed that modifying HSA NPs covalently with an appropriate PEG derivative enhances plasma circulation in vivo [32]. It shows that 5-FU-conjugated PEG-HSA-NPs were developed to improve the pharmacokinetics and therapeutic profiles of 5-FU. The findings demonstrated that the IC50 value of PEG-modified nanoparticles was considerably lower than that of unmodified nanoparticles, and the half-life was notably extended. In a similar study, the release of 5-fluorouracil from the PEGylated BSA nanoparticles was almost slower than from non-PEGylated ones, probably due to the existence of a PEG layer around PEGylated particles, which makes an extra resistance in opposition to drug diffusion.

2.4 Biocompatible, biodegradable, and safe: Low immunogenicity and nontoxic properties

Albumin is a fully biocompatible protein due to its natural presence in the body and its lack of immune response when utilized in medical applications [17, 20, 33]. It shows unique properties when interacting with biological systems, ensuring no harm, toxicity, or negative immune reactions. Hence, it has emerged as an optimal nanoparticle production and drug delivery material. Albumin is a safe and low immunogenic protein. It exhibits minimal toxicity as a naturally occurring plasma protein, rendering it safe for clinical application. Studies show that albumin isolated from pooled plasma is effective and safe for many medical applications, including plasma volume expansion, detoxification, imaging and diagnostics, coating of medical devices, and drug delivery.

Additionally, albumin is a biodegradable substance that can be metabolized in vivo into nontoxic degradation products, which the body can readily utilize or excrete. In contrast to synthetic polymers that can produce residual toxic byproducts, albumin's natural degradation pathways mitigate bioaccumulation and long-term toxicity concerns. Hence, albumin-based drug delivery is a promising strategy as it ensures safety and nontoxicity when administered at elevated doses or with repeated usage [33]. Lastly, the interaction of drugs with albumin has been shown to increase the distribution and bioavailability of the drug, influenced by the distinct pharmacokinetic characteristics of the drug molecules [18, 23, 26]. Due to its abundance, albumin strongly impacts the pharmacokinetic behavior of various drugs, including drug half-life in the bloodstream, drug efficacy regulation, drug toxicity reduction, and drug targeting specificity enhancement.

3. Mechanisms of albumin-based drug delivery

3.1 Covalent binding

In pharmacokinetic (PK) studies, the covalent bond between the drug and plasma proteins may lead to poor extraction recovery, resulting in low absorption (**Figure 1A**). Drug components can occasionally slowly separate from adducts, hindering PK and pharmacodynamic (PD) analysis. Covalent conjugation techniques

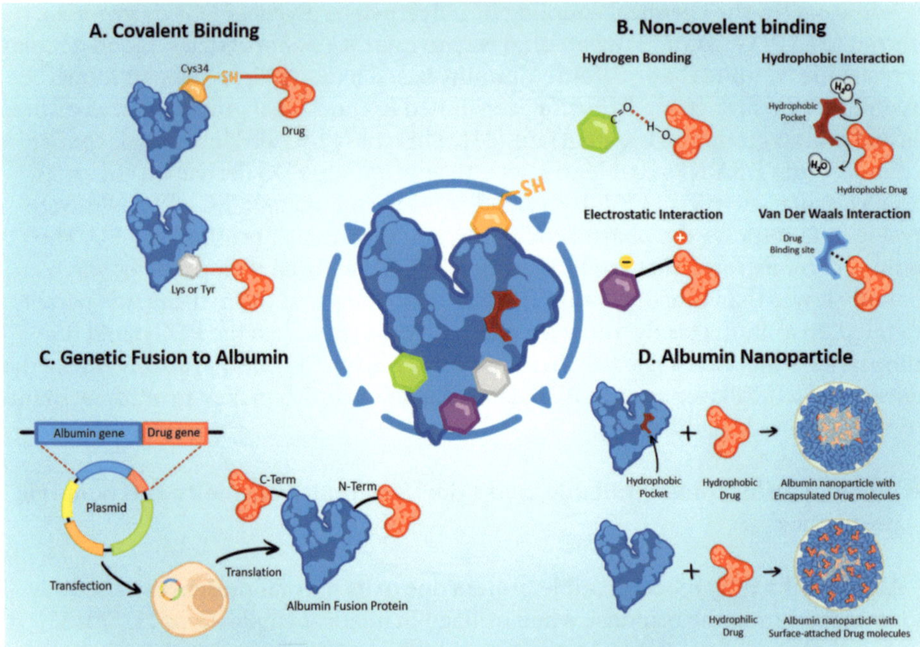

Figure 1.
Mechanisms of albumin-based drug delivery. (A) A drug of interest is covalently conjugated to either the free SH group on Cys34, lysines, or tyrosines of albumin. (B) Shows a drug binding to albumin through four different noncovalent interactions: hydrogen bonding, hydrophobic interactions, electrostatic interactions, and van der Waals forces. (C) Genetically engineered fusion protein by inserting a gene encoding a target protein at either terminus of albumin, creating a single drug construct. (D) An albumin nanoparticle with encapsulated hydrophobic drug molecules and surface-attached hydrophilic drug molecules.

are considered one of the most popular techniques used for drug control release, which are based on the albumin binding strategy [34]. For direct, covalent conjugation, the drug is typically bound to either lysines, tyrosines, or the free SH-group on the albumin residue Cys34 [35]. While albumin has 35 cysteine residues, 34 internally form disulfide bridges, which explains its exceptional stability. A free cysteine residue at position 34 for covalent drug attachment is an appealing characteristic for drug delivery since it has a free thiol group (–SH), as mentioned earlier, which makes up 80% of the thiols in plasma [36]. In addition, Cys34 is situated on the outer surface of albumin, far from the primary inner drug-binding sites; thus, it has been the focus of covalent drug conjugation [21].

Certain drugs or endogenous factors bind covalently to albumin under physiological conditions, such as acetylation of Lys199 by aspirin or glycosylation of Lys525 by D-glucose [37]. According to Meng et al. [38], Wang et al. [39], and Liu et al. [40], almost all Tyrosine Kinase Inhibitors (TKIs) can covalently bind to Lys190 of albumin. Nevertheless, Wu et al. proved that both osimertinib and furmonertinib, which are third-generation Epidermal Growth Factor Receptor (EGFR) TKIs, mainly bind to albumin through covalent bonds at Lys195 and Lys199 rather than Lys190. Another example of covalent binding is glucuronidation, a process frequently done on drugs with carboxylic acid functional groups, transforming them into acid glucuronides [41]. Acid glucuronides can covalently bond to HSA *via* two mechanisms. First, the resulting protein-drug bond is a protein-bound acyl moiety of glucuronide that can be accessed through nucleophilic attack from the protein's NH2, OH, or SH groups [34].

The other mechanism is the movement of the acyl group from position one of the sugar ring to position two, three, or four, leading to a shift in the tautomerism equilibrium of the sugar ring. In this case, the aldehyde in the open tautomer structure interacts with the lysine group inside the protein, resulting in a covalent bond between the drug and protein, with glucuronic acid binding protein [42]. In general, covalent binding to albumin will naturally impact the clearance and metabolic fate of such medications.

3.2 Noncovalent binding

On the other hand, noncovalent binding depends on weaker interactions such as hydrophobic interactions, hydrogen bonding, electrostatic interactions, and van der Waals forces (**Figure 1B**). Drug molecules can reversibly bind to albumin *via* these noncovalent interactions [43]. This type of linkage between the drug and albumin molecules is considered one of the most effective techniques for creating long-lasting biotherapeutics with enhanced PK characteristics and higher clinical performance [44]. There are many successful examples of approved medications that depend on noncovalent albumin binding. Among these are fatty acids and derivatives that led to the development of drugs like insulin detemir (Levemir®), insulin degludec (Tresiba®), liraglutide (Victoza® and Saxenda®), and semaglutide (Ozempic®), which are used to treat type 1 and 2 diabetes mellitus as well as obesity [27]. Warfarin, azapropazone, phenylbutazone, and other larger heterocyclic compounds, as well as dicarboxylic acids, are thought to attach to Sudlow Site I. On the other hand, Sudlow Site II is frequently linked to aromatic carboxylic acids, including tryptophan, ibuprofen, and diazepam [16, 45]. Ibuprofen is a nonsteroidal anti-inflammatory drug (NSAID) that has a strong affinity toward HSA. Therefore, higher doses could be needed when given in their free form to attain and sustain the intended therapeutic impact. In line with this, albumin acts as a drug reservoir; new medications are freed from binding with albumin as free drugs are eliminated from the body, extending the treatment length [46]. Additionally, albumin contains seven fatty acid binding sites distributed throughout its subdomains, which partially overlap with the two Sudlow sites previously stated, facilitating the transport of endogenous chemicals [47]. Liraglutide, for example, is a fatty acid-conjugated derivative of glucagon-like peptide-1 (GLP-1). Its albumin binding significantly extends the GLP-1 half-life after delivery from less than 2 minutes to more than 10 hours. Another noncovalent binding between drugs and albumin is electrostatic interaction, which happens when negatively charged albumin regions are drawn to positively charged drug molecule regions or vice versa. Despite being comparatively weak, the interaction aids in the drugs' binding to albumin and prolongs their circulation [48]. Lastly, hydrogen bonding occurs when a hydrogen atom in a drug molecule is covalently bound to an oxygen or nitrogen atom. This will create weak hydrogen bonds with the HSA side chain. Both the affinity of the complex and the specificity of drug binding can be enhanced by hydrogen bonding.

3.3 Fusion

Albumin fusion, which entails linking a target protein to a more stable protein, is another technology used in protein-drug development to enhance their PK properties (**Figure 1C**) [49]. Genetic engineering enables the recombinant expression of a fusion protein by inserting a gene encoding a target protein at either terminus of

HSA, creating a single drug construct with a controlled albumin-to-drug ratio [50]. Fusion proteins need to maintain their stability throughout synthesis and storage. Nevertheless, the behavior of fusion proteins cannot be predicted from the behavior of individual proteins due to their complexity and the additional intramolecular interactions. Thus, it is essential to comprehend the molecular stability of fusion proteins to produce biopharmaceuticals [50]. The function of a peptide linker is crucial for optimizing the fusion technique. A peptide linker's length and flexibility significantly impact intermolecular interactions, affecting fused proteins' in vivo biological activity. Albumin fusion technology has many advantages, and it has been proven to increase the catalytic efficiency, activity, stability, and solubility of protein drugs [51]. Additionally, it prevents rapid renal clearance by linking a target protein to a protein with a longer half-life. However, because it is difficult to anticipate the behavior of fusion proteins under different conditions, the formulation process of the fusion proteins is indeed challenging [51]. Albiglutide and Albutrepenonacog-alfa (Idelvion®, CSL Behring) are two successful examples of approved drugs that depend on an albumin-fusion strategy. The first albumin-fusion protein drug approved by the FDA is Albiglutide, used for treating patients with type 2 diabetes mellitus. It is constructed by genetically fusing two tandem modified GLP-1 molecules to the N-terminus of HSA. Albutrepenonacog-alfa (Idelvion®, CSL Behring) was approved in 2016 for treating patients with severe hemophilia B [50]. It is generated by fusing a human recombinant coagulation factor IX (rFIX) to HSA, extending the half-life beyond 100 h, five times longer than the native protein [52].

3.4 Albumin nanoparticle

Nanoparticle delivery systems have received a lot of interest as a medicine delivery method. It offers several benefits for therapeutic agents with low bioavailability and dose-limiting toxicity, including unique drug targeting, gradually controlled release properties, and a protective function, particularly in transferring hydrophobic drugs [53]. Nanotechnology is defined as a size range of around 1–100 nm, while it can be expanded to 1000 nm over a broad range (**Figure 1D**) [54]. Nevertheless, mounting evidence demonstrates that nanoparticles of sizes greater than 100 nm typically have difficulties infusing into the tumor microenvironment. Furthermore, heterogeneous distribution and intratumoral variation often hinder their deeper penetration into tissues, especially solid tumors [55].

A nanoalbumin-based drug system provides appealing benefits for overcoming the limits of conventional nanomedicines. Because albumin has many natural drug-binding sites, it easily incorporates many hydrophobic small compounds [56]. In addition, natural functional groups in albumin, such as amino and carboxylic groups and charged amino acids, can be modified with active targeting ligands *via* a cleavable linker for regulated release [6]. Furthermore, the active localization of albumin to tumors and inflammatory regions may effectively improve the penetration of albumin-based nanoparticles [57]. Several methods have been used to prepare albumin nanoparticles, e.g., desolvation, emulsification, nanoparticle albumin-bound (nab) technology, pH condensation, thermal gelation, nanospray drying, self-assembly, and microfluidic technology. Each method has its advantages and disadvantages, while the choice of the preparation technique depends on the nature of the drug, the nanoparticle characteristics needed, and the application requirements. Na Qu et al. comprehensively overview each preparation technique [20]. Nab technology is an established drug delivery platform in which albumin is used for particle stabilization. Thus, no solubilizers or emulsifiers are required during the formulation process of poorly water-soluble drugs [58]. One successful application in clinical nanomedicine based on nab technology is Abraxane® (nab-paclitaxel) [59]. It is widely used for tumor treatment, such as metastatic breast cancer [60]. Another nab technology application is Fyarro® (nab-sirolimus), which was approved for the treatment of unresectable or metastatic malignant perivascular epithelial cell tumors [58, 61]. Furthermore, in 2022, Nanozora® was approved in Japan for treating rheumatoid arthritis [20].

3.5 Albumin binding to hydrophobic and hydrophilic drugs

The solubility and stability of various drug molecules are enhanced by albumin because it can adhere to hydrophobic and hydrophilic ligands, thus improving their PK properties [13]. The characteristics of the albumin surface and drug-binding sites are particularly intriguing. In addition to having several hydrophobic binding pockets, the surface of albumin is negatively charged, which makes it highly water-soluble [4]. The primary drug-binding regions in albumin are located in the subdomains IIA and IIIA, which harbor the hydrophobic pockets Sudlow I and Sudlow II, respectively [62]. These ligand-binding pockets primarily mediate albumin binding to hydrophobic drugs [43]. The binding between the ligand and the protein is thought to involve both hydrophobic and electrostatic interactions. Sudlow I has an affinity toward warfarin, phenylbutazone, amantadine, azapropazone, azidothymidine, indomethacin, iodipamide, and oxyphenbutazone [63]. On the other hand, Sudlow II has been shown to bind with diazepam, digoxin, clofibrate, ibuprofen, benzodiazepine, halothane, propofol, and nonsteroidal anti-inflammatory drugs. When highly hydrophobic substances attach to albumin, the total solubility of the drug in plasma increases. Increased drug solubility in plasma is considered advantageous, although a high affinity for albumin will necessitate greater doses and may be a drawback [7].

3.6 The use of the albumin pathway for enhanced drug delivery

Albumin accumulation in tumors occurs through two primary mechanisms. First is the enhanced permeability and retention (EPR) effect, and second is receptor-mediated tumor internalization and catabolism [64]. The EPR effect has been extensively investigated for passive tumor targeting using macromolecular and nanoparticle therapies. While normal tissues have a dense, connected vascular endothelium through which macromolecules, including albumin, cannot easily pass except if they are transported by transcytosis [64], it has been widely documented that abnormal tumor vessels have a highly permeable architecture. Therefore, albumin and other macromolecules can freely penetrate tumor tissue and remain there for an extended period, leading to their accumulation in the tumor tissue [64]. The EPR effect depends on the intrinsic characteristics of the solid tumors, including defective blood vessels, elevated expression of inflammatory factors, and ineffective lymphatic clearance. These features enable albumin and other macromolecules to remain in the tumor tissues for an extended time [65].

In addition to the EPR effect, albumin enables active tumor targeting through receptor-mediated uptake [66]. Since albumin is a source of amino acids, the high oxygen and nutritional requirements promote overexpression of albumin-binding proteins in tumor cells, such as glycoprotein 60 (GP60) and Secreted Protein Acidic and Rich in Cysteine (SPARC). Albumin can pass through the vascular endothelial cell layer *via* binding to the GP60, expressed in the vascular endothelium. SPARC, on the other hand, is described in a variety of tumor cell types, including gliomas, liver cancer, melanoma, and breast cancer. In addition, the SPARC and Gp60 could effectively bind albumin and promote drug aggregation in tumor cells [3].

4. Applications in drug delivery

Albumin has established itself as the key carrier in nanomedicine, specifically in oncology, and this ability enhances drug delivery and its targeting. One of the successful examples of nab-paclitaxel leverage is the albumin's natural transport mechanism by improving the solubility and bioavailability of paclitaxel, a hydrophobic chemotherapeutic agent. A design enables a higher drug concentration at tumor sites while reducing systemic toxicity compared to a conventional formulation [67]. Multiple mechanisms are involved in facilitating a tumor-specific drug accumulation, including receptor-mediated endocytosis through gp60 receptors and endothelial cells that enhanced permeability and retention (EPR) effects to tumor tissues and an albumin's affinity for the SPARC (secreted protein acidic and rich in cysteine) [16, 68]. The properties enhance drug penetration across an endothelial barrier and concentrate paclitaxel in the tumor microenvironment, improving therapeutic efficacy with fewer side effects. Nab-paclitaxel reduces hypersensitivity reactions. This allows for the safe administration of higher doses [69]. Clinical applications included metastatic breast cancer, non-small lung cancer, and pancreatic cancer, where nab-paclitaxel demonstrates superior outcomes compared to a solvent-based formulation [68]. Albumin's natural role in transporting hormones, fatty acids, and different molecules makes it ideal for carrying therapeutic peptides, proteins, and small molecules. These agents often suffered limitations like low stability, short half-lives, and rapid enzymatic degradation. Albumin overcomes those challenges by forming stable complexes or covalent conjugates, and there is a significant enhancement in therapeutic efficacy [70].

For instance, tumor-targeting pesticides like BB28 and an iRGD have been combined with albumin for enhanced delivery [71]. The anticancer drug targeting bombesin receptor expression in the cancer cells was fused to an albumin-binding domain (ABD) WQRPSSW. A fusion extended a peptide's half-life in mice from 5 minutes to 2 hours. This enables better targeting of cancer cells by inducing apoptosis. Similarly, the iRGD peptide (CRGDKGPDC), which binds to the αvβ integrin receptor overexpressed in tumors, was chemically modified with cysteine to enable disulfide bonding with albumin [71]. Another notable application directly involves the stimulator of interferon genes (STING) activation, the circular pathway in the immune response. The albumin was used to create the biodegradable MnO2-albumin nanoplatforms for delivering tumor antigen peptides in STING-activating peptide nonvaccine (HAS-MnO2-pep). A system enhances the delivery of the peptides to an antigen-presenting cell (APC) and boosts an innate and adaptive immune response against tumors [72]. Albumin has also shown promise to deliver pituitary adenylate cyclase-activating peptide (PACAP), the neuropeptide involved in glucose regulation and neuroprotection [73].

For instance, MHDBAY and PACAP-derived peptide with a 7-mer albumin-binding sequence demonstrated an extended half-life of over 12 hours as compared to Exendin-4, leading to prolonged glucose control and improved therapeutic outcome in diabetes [74]. In addition, the albumin's versatility extended to antiviral applications like fusion with a CD4 to block an HIV entry into CD4+ cells, cells as the carrier for IFNβ (interferon-β) that enhance immune responses to tumor-draining lymph nodes [75]. The albumin forms a stable complex with quercetin and copper ions, enhancing quercetin's antioxidant properties while preventing oxidative degradation and its cytotoxicity.

This albumin-quercetin-Cu^{2+} complex preserves bioactivity, offering a promising approach for delivering bioactive compounds in medical and nutritional applications [76]. In diagnostics, albumin acts as an effective carrier for indocyanine green (ICG), a near-infrared fluorescent dye with phototherapeutic properties. ICG-albumin nanoparticles enhance tumor-specific accumulation, extend systemic retention, and reduce off-target toxicity, enabling precise imaging-guided cancer therapy and synergistic photodynamic/photothermal treatment [77]. Albumin-based delivery systems have significantly contributed to treating chronic diseases, including diabetes, cardiovascular diseases, rheumatoid arthritis, Alzheimer's disease, and tuberculosis. In diabetes, albumin-binding technologies have been successfully applied to antidiabetic agents like insulin analogs and glucagon-like peptide-1 (GLP-1) derivatives, as seen in products like Levemir(®) and Victoza(®) [78, 79]. Innovations such as albumin-insulin conjugates and albumin fusion proteins, including albumin, offer prolonged glucose control with reduced risk of side effects [80]. In cardiovascular diseases, albumin's application extends to improving drug targeting and delivery. For instance, milrinone, a treatment for heart failure, is conjugated with albumin to enhance myocardial contractility and cardiac function [81]. Albumin also plays a role in cardiovascular device biocompatibility by being conjugated to CD39, which reduces thrombosis risk and inflammation [82]. In rheumatoid arthritis, Ozaralizumab (Nanozora), a trivalent nanobody combining anti-TNFα and anti-HSA components, effectively neutralizes TNFα while leveraging albumin binding to extend half-life and minimize rapid clearance. This albumin-based therapy, approved in Japan in 2022, offers sustained therapeutic effects with reduced immunogenicity compared to conventional TNFα inhibitors [83]. For Alzheimer's disease, albumin-based systems combined with muco-adhesive polymers improve drug bioavailability and brain penetration for intranasal delivery, offering sustained release and enhanced therapeutic effects for drugs like meloxicam [84]. Other conditions include gout treatment with Ag-Uox (urate oxidase conjugated with albumin) to extend stability and circulation time [85]. Not to forget, albumin's potential application in managing severe COVID-19 symptoms by delivering Rg6 and Rgx365 in PEGylated albumin nanoparticles, which reduce inflammation and platelet aggregation [86]. Albumin's unique properties position it as a cornerstone in modern drug delivery and diagnostics, driving innovations that improve patient outcomes and treatment precision.

5. Advancements in albumin drug delivery technologies

5.1 Albumin nanoparticles and nanocarriers

Nanomaterials have transformed drug delivery systems, enabling innovative methods for the precise and controlled release of therapeutic agents [87]. Albumin-based nanoparticles (ABNPs) are emerging as a highly promising platform due to their biocompatibility, biodegradability, and multifunctionality [88]. A key advantage of ABNPs is their natural degradability, which lowers toxicity risks and prevents tissue accumulation [89]. Albumin, a protein naturally present in the human body, is an exceptional carrier for drug delivery. Its significant traits include the ability to bind to a wide array of molecules, such as drugs, peptides, and nucleic acids, thereby enhancing effective transport to targeted sites in the body [90]. Encapsulating these drugs within albumin nanoparticles significantly improves their solubility, leading to enhanced bioavailability and therapeutic efficacy [87]. Albumin nanoparticles serve as a cornerstone of advanced drug delivery systems due to their biocompatibility, biodegradability, and ability to enhance therapeutic efficacy [87]. Albumin, a natural transport protein, forms nanoparticles through techniques such as desolvation, emulsification, or self-assembly, enabling the encapsulation of hydrophobic drugs, such as paclitaxel or sirolimus, for improved solubility and controlled release. These nanoparticles leverage albumin's intrinsic properties, including its long circulatory half-life (~19 days), mediated by the FcRn receptor recycling, and its affinity for tumor tissues *via* the enhanced permeability and retention (EPR) effect. Recent innovations include albumin-coated nanocapsules and nanocrystals, such as atovaquone-loaded albumin nanocrystals (Ato-nCry), which demonstrated superior uptake in immune cells and melanoma cells, effectively inhibiting STAT3 phosphorylation with reduced toxicity compared to free drugs [91]. Challenges persist in fabrication methods, particularly with the use of organic solvents, which can compromise the structural integrity of albumin. Emerging solvent-free techniques and hybrid systems, such as albumin-polymer conjugates, aim to address these limitations while enhancing stability and targeting precision [92]. The functionalization of ABNPs with ligands has revolutionized targeted drug delivery, enabling precise interaction with disease-specific receptors. Albumin's surface chemistry enhances cellular uptake by allowing covalent or noncovalent modifications, such as aptamers, peptides, or antibodies. For example, AS1411 aptamer-functionalized albumin nanoparticles demonstrated increased targeting of nucleolin-overexpressing cancer cells, thereby improving doxorubicin delivery and apoptosis induction in breast cancer models [93]. In oncology, albumin nanoparticles, such as Abraxane (albumin-bound paclitaxel), utilize SPARC receptor-mediated uptake in tumors, while FcRn interactions prolong systemic circulation. Beyond cancer, these systems are explored for inflammatory diseases and gene therapy, where albumin's macropinocytosis-driven uptake in immune cells facilitates intracellular delivery of anti-inflammatory agents or CRISPR-Cas9 complexes [91]. Future directions emphasize multifunctional "theranostic" nanoparticles that combine imaging agents and therapeutics, alongside scalable fabrication methods, to accelerate clinical translation.

5.2 Preparation methods of albumin nanoparticles

Albumin nanoparticles are synthesized *via* well-established methods such as desolvation, gelation, emulsification, NAB technology, self-assembly, and spray drying, each tailored to produce specific characteristics for diverse applications in drug delivery, cancer therapy, and beyond (see **Table 1**) [104].

5.2.1 Desolvation method

The desolvation method is used for synthesizing albumin nanoparticles due to its simplicity, scalability, and ability to encapsulate both hydrophilic and hydrophobic drugs [94]. It involves gradually adding a desolating agent, such as ethanol, acetone, or methanol, to an aqueous albumin solution while stirring, thereby reducing the solubility of albumin and inducing protein aggregation into nanoparticles *via*

Method	Principle	Medication examples	Advantages	Disadvantages	Applications	Ref.
Desolvation	Adding a desolvating agent (e.g., ethanol addition) induces protein precipitation and albumin nanoparticle formation	Abraxane (paclitaxel-bound albumin nanoparticles)	Simple, controllable particle size, high drug loading (encapsulation) efficiency	The potential toxicity of desolvating agents requires stabilization Potential for protein denaturation, limited control over size and morphology	Drug delivery, diagnostics, imaging, vaccine development, theragnostic	[94, 95]
Emulsification	Formation of an emulsion followed by homogenization	Doxorubicin (CD44-targeted formulations)	Suitable for hydrophobic drugs, control over particle size and morphology, and high encapsulation efficiency	Use of organic solvents, potential for drug loss during processing	Encapsulation of hydrophobic drugs, drug delivery, imaging, and tissue engineering	[20]
Thermal gelation	Heating to denature and aggregate albumin	Curcumin (Anticancer/ Anti-inflammatory)	Simple, effective for stable nanoparticles	Limited to heat-stable drugs, potential for protein denaturation	Drug delivery, diagnostics	[6, 88]
Self-assembly	Modification to increase hydrophobicity, promoting self-assembly	Resveratrol (liver tumor targeting)	No organic solvents, stable nanoparticles	Complex modification process, limited control over particle size	Drug delivery, T-theranostics	[96]
Nab™ technology	High-pressure homogenization and desolvation	Paclitaxel (Abraxane)	High drug loading, improved therapeutic efficacy	The complex process requires specialized equipment	Cancer therapy (e.g., Abraxane)	[67, 97, 98]
Nanospray drying	Atomization and drying of albumin solution	Acyclovir (Antiviral)	Suitable for large-scale production, high drug-loading efficiency	High energy consumption, the potential for protein degradation	Dry powders for reconstitution, drug delivery	[20, 99–102]
pH coacervation	Adjusting pH to induce phase separation	Quinacrine, Fluorescent dyes Gabapentin	Encapsulates both hydrophobic and hydrophilic drugs	Sensitive to pH and ionic strength, potential for aggregation	Drug delivery, encapsulation of various drugs	[95, 103]

Method	Principle	Medication examples	Advantages	Disadvantages	Applications	Ref.
Nanoprecipitation	Mixing a protein solution with a nonsolvent induces rapid precipitation and nanoparticle formation	Thymoquinone (lung cancer therapy)	Control over particle size and morphology, high encapsulation efficiency	The potential for protein denaturation due to rapid mixing requires specialized equipment	Drug delivery, imaging, and gene therapy	[20]

Table 1.
Preparation of albumin nanoparticles.

coacervation [20, 94]. Key parameters, including pH, ionic strength, and desolvation rate, have a significant influence on particle size, drug loading, and stability. Methanol produces smaller bovine serum albumin (BSA) nanoparticles (~114 nm) due to differences in solvent polarity [94]. Post-desolvation cross-linking with glutaraldehyde or EDC stabilizes the nanoparticles, enhancing the release of the drug. This technique has successfully loaded chemotherapeutics, such as doxorubicin, thereby improving solubility and efficacy in cancer treatment. However, residual solvents pose biocompatibility challenges, prompting ongoing research into solvent optimization and the development of alternative cross-linkers. Overall, desolation remains a fundamental and adaptable method for synthesizing albumin nanoparticles in various therapeutic applications [6, 20].

5.2.2 Emulsification

The emulsification method enables precise control of albumin nanoparticle size and drug loading by forming water-in-oil emulsions, where albumin is dissolved in the aqueous phase and organic solvents containing surfactants are used, and the emulsion is stabilized using cross-linking agents like TDI. High-energy techniques, such as sonication or pressure homogenization, optimize particle uniformity, stability, and circulation time. Meanwhile, surface modifications, including PEGylation or ligand attachment, enhance tumor targeting and therapeutic efficacy. This scalable approach yields nanoparticles with high encapsulation efficiency, sustained release, and reduced systemic toxicity, rendering emulsification a versatile cornerstone for various biomedical applications [20].

5.2.3 Thermal gelation

Thermal gelation is a solvent-free, tunable method for synthesizing stable albumin nanoparticles by heating aqueous albumin solutions to induce denaturation and self-assembly through covalent bonds, such as disulfide and peptide linkages [90]. Parameters such as temperature and heating duration influence particle size, drug loading, and release profiles, with spectroscopic analyses confirming that reduced α-helical content facilitates nanoparticle formation. This technique has effectively encapsulated anticancer drugs, enhancing their efficacy and reducing toxicity in preclinical models. Despite challenges in optimizing heating protocols and scaling up production, the recent integration with microfluidic systems has enhanced reproducibility and control, establishing thermal gelation as a promising approach for future drug delivery applications [8, 105].

5.2.4 Self-assembly

The self-assembly method provides a solvent-free, biocompatible approach to synthesizing albumin nanoparticles, leveraging albumin's natural ability to form structured nanoparticles in response to environmental triggers such as temperature or pH, which involve both covalent (disulfide) and noncovalent (hydrophobic, Schiff base) interactions [6]. Elevated temperatures induce structural shifts in albumin, reducing the α-helical content and promoting cross-linking, which results in stable nanoparticles with controlled drug release. This is especially beneficial for hydrophobic drugs, such as anticancer agents, which achieve high encapsulation efficiency and reduced toxicity. These nanoparticles degrade predictably under enzymatic or reductive conditions, allowing for customizable release profiles [90, 106]. Albumin's innate targeting *via* gp60 receptors enhances tumor accumulation through the EPR effect, exemplified by clinical use in nab-paclitaxel (Abraxane). Recent surface modifications, such as PEGylation or ligand attachment, further enhance targeting and circulation, making self-assembly a scalable and biodegradable platform for advanced albumin-based nanomedicines [6].

5.2.5 Nab™ technology (high-pressure homogenization)

Nab™ (nanoparticle albumin-bound) technology is an innovative platform for creating stable, biocompatible albumin nanoparticles that enhance the delivery and efficacy of hydrophobic drugs like chemotherapeutics without toxic solvents or emulsifiers [67]. It involves dissolving drugs, such as paclitaxel, in organic solvents and emulsifying with aqueous albumin under high shear forces, often using a Microfluidizer, to produce uniform nanoparticles (~130 nm). This is followed by solvent removal, sterilization, and lyophilization for intravenous use. Albumin's natural ability to bind receptors, such as gp60 on endothelial cells, facilitates targeted tumor delivery *via* the EPR effect, thereby improving drug solubility, bioavailability, and patient tolerance, as exemplified by the FDA-approved Abraxane for various cancers [67, 88]. The platform's versatility extends to other poorly soluble drugs, such as itraconazole, making Nab™ a scalable, effective, and safer nanomedicine approach for cancer and beyond [67].

5.2.6 pH coacervation

The pH-coacervation method is an efficient, scalable technique for producing biocompatible albumin nanoparticles by adjusting pH to induce protein aggregation, enabling effective drug encapsulation and controlled release [95]. It enables precise particle size tuning through parameters such as desolvation rate and cross-linker strength, with applications demonstrated in the sustained delivery of drugs like quinacrine and gabapentin, which exhibit prolonged release and enhanced brain targeting. Surface modifications, such as polysorbate 80 coating, further enhance efficacy, as exemplified by increased drug accumulation in the brain for epilepsy treatment. This solvent-free approach is suitable for both hydrophilic and hydrophobic drugs, making it a versatile and scalable platform for developing albumin-based nanocarriers for cancer, neurological, and other diseases [95].

5.2.7 Nanoprecipitation

The nanoprecipitation method is a simple and scalable approach for synthesizing albumin nanoparticles that effectively encapsulate both hydrophilic and hydrophobic drugs, eliminating the need for toxic solvents. Key parameters, including BSA concentration, pH, and solvent ratio, influence particle size, stability, and drug loading [107]. Recent advances include microfluidic systems that improve control, reduce particle size by 15–20%, and enhance reproducibility. This technique yields biocompatible nanoparticles with high encapsulation efficiency (e.g., ~82% for paclitaxel) and sustained release, leveraging albumin's natural affinity for receptors like gp60 to promote tumor targeting *via* the EPR effect, as seen in FDA-approved Abraxane [106]. Despite challenges in polydispersity control, ongoing optimization of process parameters continues to improve its clinical potential, making nanoprecipitation a versatile and cost-effective strategy for albumin-based nanocarriers [20, 107].

5.2.8 Spray drying

Spray drying is a scalable, solvent-free technique for producing uniform albumin nanoparticles with high yields (>70%), ideal for pulmonary delivery and targeting applications [108]. It involves atomizing albumin solutions into fine droplets, rapidly drying them with heated air to create stable, spherical nanoparticles, further enhanced by PEGylation or lipid conjugation for improved stability and release profiles [108]. This method effectively encapsulates heat-sensitive therapeutics, such as acyclovir, achieving high encapsulation efficiencies and deep lung penetration while avoiding toxic organic solvents and simplifying purification. Albumin's natural receptor-mediated targeting, such as gp60 binding, synergizes with spray-dried formulations to enhance tumor accumulation and localized delivery in infections and cancer [66, 92]. Despite challenges such as particle aggregation, ongoing process optimizations and innovative nozzle designs continue to establish spray drying as a cornerstone for industrial-scale albumin nanomedicine production, enabling versatile applications ranging from inhalable therapies to targeted drug delivery [66, 92].

5.3 Albumin nanoparticle modification for enhanced drug delivery

Albumin nanoparticles (ABNPs) play a crucial role in nanomedicine due to their biocompatibility and biodegradability, making them ideal carriers for targeted drug delivery. Current research has focused on modifying these nanoparticles to optimize their functional properties, with surface functionalization and conjugation being key strategies [20]. Derived from sources such as human, bovine, or egg albumin, these nanocarriers exploit albumin's natural affinity for specific cell receptors, including gp60, thereby promoting tumor targeting through the enhanced permeability and retention (EPR) effect [106]. To further improve their performance, chemical modifications such as PEGylation (the attachment of polyethylene glycol) are employed to increase stability and extend systemic circulation by reducing immune clearance. Additionally, conjugation with ligands such as folic acid, hyaluronic acid, or transferrin enables the active targeting of cancer cells that overexpress specific receptors, thereby addressing challenges such as nonspecific drug distribution and the limitations of unmodified nanoparticles [109]. These innovations have made albumin nanoparticles a pivotal component in the development of advanced drug delivery platforms, with broad therapeutic applications in oncology and beyond. In parallel, the unique physical properties, controllable structures, and surface chemistries of metal and inorganic nanoparticles provide significant advantages in biomedical applications, especially in antimicrobial and antitumor therapies. Metal nanoparticles such as gold, silver, and copper are widely used to inhibit bacterial growth and enhance the efficacy of chemotherapy, often complementing radiation therapy. Magnetic nanoparticles, such as Fe3O4, facilitate targeted drug delivery, particularly when combined with albumin to form inorganic-albumin hybrid systems [110]. Biomineralization combines albumin's high hydrophilicity, multiple binding sites, and reduction capabilities with the beneficial properties of inorganic materials, thereby boosting therapeutic outcomes in photothermal therapy and immunotherapy. Recent developments in albumin-magnetic nanoparticles (AMNPs) have significantly enhanced targeted cancer treatment by leveraging albumin's natural drug-binding capacity, along with its magnetic properties, to achieve higher delivery efficiency and specificity [111]. Despite their promise, challenges persist in scalability and batch consistency; however, innovations such as microfluidic fabrication and spray drying are addressing these issues. Future directions focus on multifunctional hybrid systems, including albumin-metal nanocomposites for combined therapy and imaging, as well as stimuli-responsive nanoparticles designed to release drugs in response to pH or enzymatic triggers, broadening the horizons for safer, more personalized treatments in nanomedicine [20, 110].

5.3.1 Engineered albumin variants and albumin-drug conjugates

5.3.1.1 Engineered albumin variants for enhanced targeting

Engineered albumin variants are modified forms of the protein designed to overcome the limitations of native albumin, such as limited drug-loading capacity, reliance on passive targeting, and instability in challenging environments [112]. Engineered variants such as Veltis High Binder II (HBII) exhibit an enhanced affinity for the neonatal Fc receptor (FcRn) [112]. This improved binding translates to a longer circulation time and more significant tumor drug accumulation *via* FcRn-mediated recycling. Consequently, this modification enables a consistent release of drugs within the tumor microenvironment, as shown by studies with conjugates that release monomethyl auristatin E (MMAE) in vivo [112]. The cysteine-34 residue of albumin is often targeted for structural modifications due to its accessibility. Carbonylacrylic (caa) reagents facilitate a stable and reliable attachment of drugs while preserving FcRn binding, which is essential for maintaining pharmacokinetic benefits. Additionally, protease-responsive linkers, such as valine-citrulline [VC(S)], serve as cleavable linkers that utilize tumor-associated proteases, like cathepsin B, to release cytotoxic agents, such as MMAE. These linkers enable selective drug activation within tumors, thereby minimizing off-target toxicity. Genetic engineering in protein production, such as recombinant albumin, is produced using yeast (Pichia pastoris) or bacterial systems, eliminating batch variability and addressing ethical concerns related to animal-derived proteins [3]. A notable example is Recombumin, developed by Novozymes, used in FDA-approved medications like Abraxane (nab-paclitaxel) [67]. Adding cysteine residues at certain locations, particularly at position 34, enables targeted drug conjugation. This leads to the creation of Cys34-modified human serum albumin (HSA), which supports the covalent attachment of paclitaxel, enhancing its tumor accumulation and stability of the payload. Furthermore, mutations within albumin's FcRn-binding domain significantly extend its circulatory half-life beyond the native approximately 19 days [112]. These modifications are essential for prolonged circulation and crucial for effective drug delivery.

5.3.1.2 Albumin-drug conjugation strategies

Albumin-drug conjugation strategies are crucial for improving therapeutic efficacy by utilizing albumin's natural traits, such as its extended circulation half-life, biocompatibility, and ability to target *via* receptors. **Table 2** shows the key methods, along with their mechanisms and uses.

5.3.2. Innovations in albumin-bound imaging agents for diagnostics

Albumin's unique structural and functional characteristics, including biocompatibility, a prolonged circulation half-life, and an inherent affinity for tumor-associated receptors, have driven its use in the development of advanced imaging agents. These

Strategy	Mechanism	Examples/uses
Covalent conjugation	Glutaraldehyde cross-linking (Schiff base), EDC/NHS (amide bonds), disulfide bonding (thiol groups)	Doxorubicin-albumin for breast cancer, methotrexate-albumin for RA, camptothecin-albumin for colon cancer [113–115]
Noncovalent conjugation	Hydrophobic interactions (Sudlow sites), electrostatic interactions (siRNA binding), lipid binding with ethylene glycol linkers	Abraxane (paclitaxel) for breast/pancreatic cancer, albumin-siRNA for TNBC and hepatocellular carcinoma [116, 117]
Prodrug strategies	Fatty acid-mediated conjugation (PEG-lipid anchors), enzyme-cleavable linkers (peptide/ester)	Doxorubicin prodrug for tumor targeting, gemcitabine-albumin for pancreatic cancer [114]
Hybrid systems	Ligand-modified conjugates (folate, RGD), dual-drug conjugation (albumin nanoparticles)	Folate-albumin-paclitaxel for ovarian cancer, albumin-cisplatin-gemcitabine for lung cancer [118]

Table 2.
Albumin-drug conjugation strategies.

breakthroughs enhance diagnostic accuracy, enable multimodal imaging, and integrate theragnostic features. Below are significant advancements in albumin-bound imaging agents for diagnostics, categorized by modality and application (**Table 3**). Challenges in albumin nanoparticle development include synthesis complexity, where organic solvents can disrupt albumin structure, and variability in tumor receptor expression, necessitating personalized profiling [92]. Conjugation chemistry significantly impacts toxicity and biodistribution, influencing off-target organ uptake (e.g., the lungs) and risks such as thrombocytopenia, highlighting the need for opsonin-resistant designs [118]. Transitioning to clinical use requires formulations with improved stability, scalability, and regulatory approval, exemplified by FDA-approved drugs like Abraxane [121]. Emerging approaches such as albumin-cell conjugates for immune evasion and stimuli-responsive nanoparticles for controlled drug release offer promising avenues to enhance safety and efficacy. Ongoing research is crucial for optimizing nanoparticle design to achieve safe and effective cancer diagnostics and therapy [125].

5.4 Strategies to mitigate protein aggregation

There are several ways to mitigate protein aggregation. For example, detergents and amphiphiles, such as ionic surfactants and anionic surfactants, as well as phospholipid vesicles and surfactants, might affect protein aggregation. Cyclodextrins, which are circular glucose-based polymers, have shown potential in inhibiting protein aggregation by binding aromatic residues, stabilizing unfolded states, and slowing folding rates. They have been used to prevent aggregation in therapeutic proteins and as chaperones for protein refolding. Lyophilization, or freeze-drying, usually extends protein shelf life by removing water through vacuum sublimation. While low temperatures generally preserve proteins, multiple freeze cycles can induce aggregation by creating nucleation sites at ice-water interfaces, altering pH, and causing phase separation. Hence, it is essential to properly control lyophilization parameters, such as formulation composition and drying conditions [126]. Other attempts to solve aggregation issues have been made with the use of computational methods to identify

Focus area	Key insights and significance	Examples and features	Ref.
Enhanced relaxivity MRI contrast agents	• Significantly improve MRI resolution and safety • Surpass traditional gadolinium agents Use passive (EPR) and active (receptor) targeting mechanisms	• Gadolinium complexes and iron oxide nanoparticles • Exploit the EPR effect for passive targeting Receptor pathways *via* GP60 and SPARC for active targeting	[92]
Nuclear imaging probes for tumor targeting	• Extend the circulation time of radiotracers • Increase tumor retention and contrast Enable clearer PET/SPECT imaging for therapy monitoring	• PET and SPECT tracers • Stable tumor uptake (2.7–3.8% ID/cm^3) • High tumor/muscle ratios (3.2–9.4) e.g. [68Ga] Ga-L6, [177Lu] Lu-L6, 111In-C4-DTPA	[119] [120]
Optical imaging with programmable probes	• Reduce background signals and photobleaching • Enable real-time tumor margin visualization Facilitate dual-wavelength imaging for diagnosis and therapy	• Cyanine-Albumin with IPBA • NIR-II dyes (IR825) with aggregation-induced emission Dual-wavelength imaging (600 nm and 808 nm) for the separation of imaging and therapy	[121] [122]
Theragnostic platforms for combined imaging and therapy	• Achieve complete tumor eradication • Combine diagnosis with targeted photothermal and radiotherapy Improve safety through renal clearance	• Fluorescence-guided photothermal ablation (HSA-IR825) • Dual-targeting radiotracers (FAPI-RGD) enhance PET/CT imaging and radionuclide therapy, especially for lung cancer. Effective in murine models	[122] [119, 123]
Receptor-mediated targeting mechanisms	• Exploit tumor receptors (GP60, SPARC) for targeted delivery • Enhance imaging contrast and treatment efficacy • Increase tumor uptake 2–3 times in high-SPARC tumors	• GP60 facilitates crossing endothelial barriers (blood vessels) • SPARC increases tumor uptake (2–3x) Applications include Abraxane and cisplatin-loaded nanoparticles	[13, 111] [124]

Table 3.
Overview of innovations in albumin-bound imaging agents for diagnostics.

the hotspots in the sequence [127]. Various strategies have been investigated to inhibit HSA aggregation, encompassing both naturally occurring small molecules and synthetically designed compounds. Natural inhibitors include simple bioactive molecules that interact with HSA to prevent its aggregation, while synthetic approaches involve the development of engineered compounds, such as nanoparticles, that can modulate protein stability and aggregation pathways. Some naturally occurring metabolites have been demonstrated to be able to inhibit fibrillation; these are sugars such as fructose, ribose, and sucrose. The ThT binding study, circular dichroism, and turbidity assay demonstrate that fructose is the most efficient inhibitor of HSA fibrillation [128].

In another study, they explored the effect of three synthesized amphiphilic surface active ionic liquids (SAILs), namely 1-methyl-3-octyl imidazolium chloride ([C 8 mim] Cl), 1-dodecyl-3-methyllimidazolium chloride ([C 12 mim] Cl), and 1-hexadecyl-3-methyllimidazolium chloride ([C16 mim] Cl) on bovine serum albumin (BSA) and human serum albumin (HSA) fibril. These SAILs have different alkyl chain lengths attached to the cationic imidazolium headgroups. Interestingly, it is observed that all three SAILs exhibit fibril inhibition at room temperature [105]. Additionally, nanoparticles have shown promising results in the inhibition of aggregation; for example, the effect of graphene oxide (GO) nanoparticles on serum albumin (HSA) was studied, and it is shown that GO interacts strongly with HSA. This is possible through different nonbonding forces like aromatic interactions, hydrogen bonding, hydrophobic and electrostatic interactions, and so forth. Such interactions can prevent the interactions between the HSA molecules upon incubation with GO. From ThT fluorescence spectroscopy, it was evident that the extent of formation of fibrillar structures of HSA is decreased [129]. Another study to be mentioned used specific magnetic nanoparticles (MNP), which are being explored increasingly in bio-related applications due to their magnetic properties, biocompatibility, and relative nontoxicity, with modifications that act on the protein assembly. An effective MNP inhibition of HSA aggregates was found in the presence of aminated magnetic $MnFe_2O_4$ nanoparticles, which was demonstrated to be effective by ThT fluorescence spectroscopy, circular dichroism, and transmission electron microscopy [130].

6. Challenges and limitations

While albumin offers numerous advantages in drug application, several challenges and limitations need to be addressed to optimize its performance. Key issues include the stability of the albumin-drug complex, the potential of drug-drug interactions, and scalability and manufacturing. Cellular geometry influences uptake efficiency; larger cancer cells like MCF-7 and A549 show enhanced micelle uptake, while normal fibroblasts with greater spreading areas exhibit reduced uptake (**Figure 2A**) [131]. Albumin's net negative charge at physiological pH may limit drug loading, though this can be improved by functionalizing with carboxyl, hydroxyl, or amino groups [133]. Environmental factors such as pH shifts can induce reversible conformational change affecting the drug release [132]. Oxidative and reductive modifications, particularly at the cysteine and methionine residues, along with chemical degradation (deamination, truncation, and hydrolysis), impair albumin's stability and binding capacity (**Figure 2B**) [134]. The use of cross-linkers to stabilize albumin nanoparticles may introduce toxicity and compromise drug efficacy [135]. Additionally, the limitations of the EPR effect (heterogeneous vascular hyperpermeability, poor cellular uptake post-extravasation, and passive targeting) necessitate active targeting strategies to enhance specificity and efficacy [136]. For albumin-nucleic acid complexes, rapid nuclease degradation in serum limits their stability and in vivo use [137]. On the other hand, albumin's use in drug delivery is challenged by drug-drug interactions due to its structural flexibility and multiple binding sites (**Figure 2C**). While albumin has two primary drug-binding sites, additional sites may be revealed, leading to potential competition or interference [138]. Different binding sites allow simultaneous binding or concurrent interactions that may influence their therapeutic outcomes. High-affinity drugs may displace others, altering their distribution and efficacy [63]. This competition can change pharmacokinetics, clearance rates, and

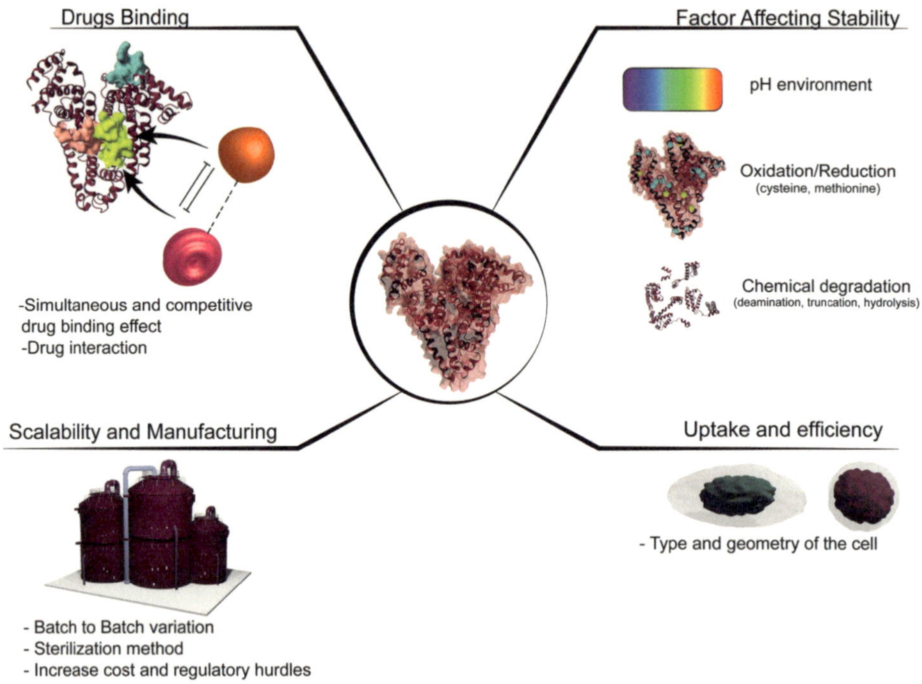

Figure 2.
Key challenges in albumin-based drug delivery. Schematic representation outlines the major challenges associated with albumin in drug delivery, categorized into four key areas: (A) Uptake and efficiency, influenced by cell type and geometry. (B) Factors affecting stability, affected by pH, oxidation/reduction, and chemical degradation. (C) Drug binding, competitive, and simultaneous drug interactions alter pharmacokinetics. (D) Scalability and manufacturing challenges include batch variability, sterilization, and regulatory hurdles.

tissue distribution, leading to unexpected therapeutic outcomes or toxicity. Moreover, coadministered drugs may interact with albumin-bound molecules, causing synergistic or antagonistic effects, complicating their use as a predictable drug [63]. The scalability and manufacturing of albumin-based drug delivery systems face key challenges for clinical application (**Figure 2D**). Batch-to-batch variability affects the consistency and drug delivery properties, complicating large-scale production [139]. Sterilization methods like heat and radiation can also compromise the albumin-drug complex, requiring alternatives to preserve its integrity [140]. Additionally, producing high-quality, pharmaceutical-grade albumin is costly, limiting its widespread use [2]. Despite some regulatory approvals, extensive clinical trials remain necessary, delaying manufacturing [88]. Addressing these challenges is critical for clinical integration and requires continued research in nanomedicine. Another significant challenge in the development of albumin-based drugs is their inherent instability, particularly protein aggregation, which raises biopharmaceutical quality concerns due to its potential to trigger immunogenic responses and antidrug antibodies (ADA) formation [141]. To mitigate these risks, optimizing protein sequences, formulations, containers, and storage conditions is essential [142]. Protein aggregation can result from stresses during manufacturing, transportation, and administration, including mechanical impacts [143]. The primary factors influencing albumin denaturation include high temperature and pH, which disrupt noncovalent interactions critical for stability. Additionally, the presence of alcohol as a cosolvent also promotes protein aggregation [144]. A recent study showed that HSA incubated at 37°C and pH 2.0

for 7–9 days formed fibrils and β-structural aggregates (not present in native HSA), increasing hydrophobicity surrounding Sudlow's sites I and II and reducing ligand binding. Partial exposure of hydrophobic residues initiates cross-linking, impairing drug transport capacity [145]. BSA aggregation was also found to vary with pH values between 4.7 and 6.2 and temperatures between 50 and 80°C, forming an amyloid fibril structure at pH above pI. Mechanistic methods can be used to identify and differentiate nanoparticle structures in aggregation. Temperature and pH may alter the size of BSA-based nanoparticles and the rate of aggregation [145]. Electrostatic interactions influence HSA fibrillation, as shown by spectroscopic studies under varying pH, temperature, and ionic strength. At physiological pH, up to 50 mM NaCl promotes fibril formation by electrostatic shielding, while higher concentrations inhibit it. In contrast, under acidic conditions, increasing salt concentration consistently enhances HSA fibrillation [145].

7. Conclusion

Albumin serves as an effective drug delivery carrier because of biocompatibility, extended circulatory half-life, and ligand-binding capabilities. This chapter examined an albumin's role in the transportation of drugs and emphasized its applications in a nanoparticle formulation for controlling drug release and targeted therapy. Various preparation techniques like optimization of albumin nanoparticles, oncology, diabetes, and neurogenerative disease. The advances in engineering albumin variants and albumin drug conjugates further improve drug stability and targeting. Despite the challenges in stability and larger-scale manufacturing, albumin's adaptability in nanomedicine makes it a cornerstone for future pharmaceutical innovation, promising enhanced treatment precision with reduced toxicity.

Acknowledgements

We would like to thank King Abdullah University of Science and Technology for financial support.

Conflict of interest

The authors declare no conflict of interest.

Disclaimer

The views expressed in this paper are those of the author(s) and do not necessarily reflect those of the SFDA or its stakeholders. Guaranteeing the accuracy and validity of the data is the sole responsibility of the research team.

Author details

Samah Al-Harthi[1†*], Awatef Alshehri[2†], Lubna Alhudhali[3], Mawadda Alghrably[3], Giulia Bennici[3], Maram Almohaywi[1], Łukasz Jaremko[3] and Mariusz Jaremko[3*]

1 Saudi Food and Drug Authority, Riyadh, Saudi Arabia

2 Department of Nanomedicine, King Abdullah International Medical Research Center (KAIMRC), King Saud bin Abdelaziz University for Health Sciences (KSAU-HS), Ministry of National Guard-Health Affairs (MNGHA), Riyadh, Saudi Arabia

3 Bioscience Program, Division of Biological and Environmental Sciences and Engineering, King Abdullah University of Science and Technology, Thuwal, Saudi Arabia

*Address all correspondence to: smharthi@sfda.gov.sa
and mariusz.jaremko@kaust.edu.sa

†These author contributed equally.

References

[1] Al-Harthi S, Lachowicz JI, Nowakowski ME, Jaremko M, Jaremko Ł. Towards the functional high-resolution coordination chemistry of blood plasma human serum albumin. Journal of Inorganic Biochemistry. 2019;**198**:110716

[2] Ashraf S, Qaiser H, Tariq S, Khalid A, Makeen HA, Alhazmi HA, et al. Unraveling the versatility of human serum albumin–A comprehensive review of its biological significance and therapeutic potential. Current Research in Structural Biology. 2023;**6**:100114

[3] Larsen MT, Kuhlmann M, Hvam ML, Howard KA. Albumin-based drug delivery: Harnessing nature to cure disease. Molecular and Cellular Therapies. 2016;**4**(1):1-12

[4] Peters Jr T. All About Albumin: Biochemistry, Genetics, and Medical Applications. 1st ed. Boston, MA: Academic Press; 1995. 432 p. DOI: 10.1016/B978-012552110-9/50006-4

[5] Levitt DG, Levitt MD. Human serum albumin homeostasis: A new look at the roles of synthesis, catabolism, renal and gastrointestinal excretion, and the clinical value of serum albumin measurements. International Journal of General Medicine. 2016;**9**:229-255

[6] Elzoghby AO, Samy WM, Elgindy NA. Albumin-based nanoparticles as potential controlled release drug delivery systems. Journal of Controlled Release. 2012;**157**:168-182

[7] Fasano M, Curry S, Terreno E, Galliano M, Fanali G, Narciso P, et al. The extraordinary ligand binding properties of human serum albumin. IUBMB Life. 2005;**57**:787-796

[8] Fujiwara S, Amisaki T. Fatty acid binding to serum albumin: Molecular simulation approaches. Biochimica et Biophysica Acta (BBA)-General Subjects. 2013;**1830**(12):5427-5434

[9] Sugio S, Kashima A, Mochizuki S, Noda M, Kobayashi K. Crystal structure of human serum albumin at 2.5 Å resolution. Protein Engineering. 1999;**12**(6):439-446

[10] Fahy KM, Eiken MK, Baumgartner KV, Leung KQ, Anderson SE, Berggren E, et al. Silver nanoparticle surface chemistry determines interactions with human serum albumin and cytotoxic responses in human liver cells. ACS Omega. 2023;**8**(3):3310-3318

[11] Garcovich M, Zocco MA, Gasbarrini A. Clinical use of albumin in hepatology. Blood Transfusion. 2009;**7**(4):268

[12] Raoufinia R, Mota A, Keyhanvar N, Safari F, Shamekhi S, Abdolalizadeh J. Overview of albumin and its purification methods. Advanced Pharmaceutical Bulletin. 2016;**6**(4):495

[13] Bhushan B, Khanadeev V, Khlebtsov B, Khlebtsov N, Gopinath P. Impact of albumin based approaches in nanomedicine: Imaging, targeting and drug delivery. Advances in Colloid and Interface Science. 2017;**246**:13-39

[14] Hutapea TPH, Madurani KA, Syahputra MY, Hudha MN, Asriana AN, Suprapto, et al. Albumin: Source, preparation, determination, applications, and prospects. Journal of Science: Advanced Materials and Devices. 2023;**8**:100549

[15] Pathania A. Chemistry behind serum albumin: A review. E3S Web of Conferences. 2021;**309**:01086

[16] Spada A, Emami J, Tuszynski JA, Lavasanifar A. The uniqueness of albumin as a carrier in nanodrug delivery. Molecular Pharmaceutics. 2021;**18**(5):1862-1894

[17] Sleep D. Albumin and its application in drug delivery. Expert Opinion on Drug Delivery. Informa Healthcare. 2015;**12**:793-812

[18] Ankita V, Priyankar S, Ejaz A, Mohd R, Naidu S, Hasan KR. Ligand binding strategies of human serum albumin: How can the cargo be utilized? Chirality. 2009;**22**(1):77-87. DOI: 10.1002/chir.20709

[19] Mauro F, Stephen C, Enzo T, Monica G, Gabriella F, Pasquale N, et al. The extraordinary ligand binding properties of human serum albumin. IUBMB Life. 2008;**57**(12):787-796. DOI: 10.1080/15216540500404093

[20] Qu N, Song K, Ji Y, Liu M, Chen L, Lee RJ, et al. Albumin nanoparticle-based drug delivery systems. International Journal of Nanomedicine. 2024;**19**:6945-6980

[21] Kratz F. Albumin as a drug carrier: Design of prodrugs, drug conjugates and nanoparticles. Journal of Controlled Release. 2008;**132**(3):171-183

[22] Carter DC, He XM. Structure of human serum albumin. Science. 1990;**249**:302-303

[23] Kragh-Hansen U. Structure and ligand binding properties of human serum albumin. Danish Medical Bulletin. 1990;**37**:57-84

[24] Lee P, Wu X. Review: Modifications of human serum albumin and their binding effect. Current Pharmaceutical Design. 2015;**21**(14):1862-1865

[25] Bujacz A. Structures of bovine, equine and leporine serum albumin. Acta Crystallographica. Section D, Biological Crystallography. 2012;**68**(10):1278-1289

[26] Sudlow G, Birkett DJ, Wade DN. The characterization of two specific drug binding sites on human serum albumin. Molecular Pharmacology. 1975;**11**(6):824-832. Available from: http://molpharm.aspetjournals.org/content/11/6/824.abstract

[27] Sleep D, Cameron J, Evans LR. Albumin as a versatile platform for drug half-life extension. Biochimica et Biophysica Acta - General Subjects. 2013;**1830**:5526-5534

[28] Aguilera-Garrido A, del Castillo-Santaella T, Yang Y, Galisteo-González F, Gálvez-Ruiz MJ, Molina-Bolívar JA, et al. Applications of serum albumins in delivery systems: Differences in interfacial behaviour and interacting abilities with polysaccharides. Advances in Colloid and Interface Science. 2021;**290**:102365

[29] Taguchi K, Giam Chuang VT, Maruyama T, Otagiri M. Pharmaceutical aspects of the recombinant human serum albumin dimer: Structural characteristics, biological properties, and medical applications. Journal of Pharmaceutical Sciences. 2012;**101**(9):3033-3046. Available from: http://www.sciencedirect.com/science/article/pii/S0022354915314490

[30] Knudsen Sand KM, Bern M, Nilsen J, Noordzij HT, Sandlie I, Andersen JT. Unraveling the interaction between FcRn and albumin: Opportunities for design of albumin-based therapeutics. Frontiers in Immunology. 2015;**6**:118912

[31] Kouchakzadeh H, Shojaosadati SA, Maghsoudi A, Vasheghani Farahani E.

Optimization of PEGylation conditions for BSA nanoparticles using response surface methodology. AAPS PharmSciTech. 2010;**11**(3):1206-1211

[32] Fahrländer E, Schelhaas S, Jacobs A, Langer K. PEGylated human serum albumin (HSA) nanoparticles: Preparation, characterization and quantification of the PEGylation extent. Nanotechnology. 2015;**26**:145103

[33] Zwain T, Zwayen S, Singh KK, Taneja N, Shidhaye A, Palshetkar A. Albumin nanoparticles—A versatile and a safe platform for drug delivery applications. In: Nanoparticle Therapeutics: Production Technologies, Types of Nanoparticles, and Regulatory Aspects. Amsterdam, The Netherlands: Elsevier; 2022. pp. 327-358

[34] Wu Y, Chen L, Chen J, Xue H, He Q, Zhong D, et al. Covalent binding mechanism of furmonertinib and osimertinib with human serum albumin. Drug Metabolism and Disposition. 2023;**51**(1):8-16

[35] Wu B, Melhem M, Subramanian R, Chen P, Jaramilla Sloey B, Fouqueray B, et al. Clinical pharmacokinetics and pharmacodynamics of etelcalcetide, a novel calcimimetic for treatment of secondary hyperparathyroidism in patients with chronic kidney disease on hemodialysis. The Journal of Clinical Pharmacology. 2018;**58**(6):717-726. DOI: 10.1002/jcph.1090

[36] Quinlan G, Martin G, Evans T. Albumin: Biochemical properties and therapeutic potential. Hepatology. 2005;**41**:1211-1219

[37] Ascoli G, Domenici E, Bertucci C. Drug binding to human serum albumin: Abridged review of results obtained with high-performance liquid chromatography and circular dichroism. Chirality. 2006;**18**:667-679

[38] Meng J, Zhang H, Bao JJ, Chen ZD, Liu XY, Zhang YF, et al. Metabolic disposition of the EGFR covalent inhibitor furmonertinib in humans. Acta Pharmacologica Sinica. 2022;**43**(2):494-503

[39] Wang J, Li-Chan X, Atherton J, Deng L, Espina R, Yu L, et al. Characterization of HKI-272 covalent binding to human serum albumin. Drug Metabolism and Disposition. 2010;**38**:1083-1093

[40] Liu X, Feng D, Zheng M, Cui Y, Zhong D. Characterization of covalent binding of tyrosine kinase inhibitors to plasma proteins. Drug Metabolism and Pharmacokinetics. 2020;**35**(5):456-465. Available from: https://www.sciencedirect.com/science/article/pii/S1347436720303992

[41] Yang G, Ge S, Singh R, Basu S, Shatzer K, Zen M, et al. Glucuronidation: Driving factors and their impact on glucuronide disposition. Drug Metabolism Reviews. 2017;**49**:105-138

[42] Kragh-Hansen U, Chuang V, Otagiri M. Practical aspects of the ligand-binding and enzymatic properties of human serum albumin. Biological & Pharmaceutical Bulletin. 2002;**25**:695-704

[43] Wu B, Wang J, Chen Y, Fu Y. Inflammation-targeted drug delivery strategies via albumin-based systems. ACS Biomaterials Science & Engineering. 2024;**10**(2):743-761

[44] Zorzi A, Linciano S, Angelini A. Non-covalent albumin-binding ligands for extending the circulating half-life of small biotherapeutics. MedChemComm. 2019;**10**:1068-1081

[45] Yamasaki K, Chuang VTG, Maruyama T, Otagiri M. Albumin–drug interaction and its clinical implication. Biochimica et Biophysica Acta (BBA) - General Subjects. 2013;**1830**(12):5435-5443. Available from: https://www.sciencedirect.com/science/article/pii/S0304416513002018

[46] Ploch-Jankowska A, Pentak D, Nycz JE. A comprehensive spectroscopic analysis of the ibuprofen binding with human serum albumin, part II. Scientia Pharmaceutica. 2021;**89**(3):30

[47] Linciano S, Moro G, Zorzi A, Angelini A. Molecular analysis and therapeutic applications of human serum albumin-fatty acid interactions. Journal of Controlled Release. 2022;**348**:115-126

[48] Lau CYJ, Benne N, Lou B, Zharkova O, Ting HJ, Ter Braake D, et al. Modulating albumin-mediated transport of peptide-drug conjugates for antigen-specific Treg induction. Journal of Controlled Release. 2022;**348**:938-950

[49] Schulte S. Innovative coagulation factors: Albumin fusion technology and recombinant single-chain factor VIII. Thrombosis Research. 2013;**131**:S2-S6. Available from: https://www.sciencedirect.com/science/article/pii/S0049384813701506

[50] Rahimizadeh P, Yang S, Lim SI. Albumin: An emerging opportunity in drug delivery. Biotechnology and Bioprocess Engineering. 2020;**25**:985-995

[51] Yang H, Liu L, Xu F. The promises and challenges of fusion constructs in protein biochemistry and enzymology. Applied Microbiology and Biotechnology. 2016;**100**:8273-8281

[52] Chia J, Louber J, Glauser I, Taylor S, Bass GT, Dower SK, et al. Half-life–extended recombinant coagulation factor IX–albumin fusion protein is recycled via the FcRn-mediated pathway. Journal of Biological Chemistry. 2018;**293**(17):6363-6373

[53] Rizvi SAA, Saleh AM. Applications of nanoparticle systems in drug delivery technology. Saudi Pharmaceutical Journal. 2018;**26**(1):64-70

[54] Bharali DJ, Khalil M, Gurbuz M, Simone TM, Mousa SA. Nanoparticles and cancer therapy: A concise review with emphasis on dendrimers. International Journal of Nanomedicine. 2009;**4**:1-7

[55] Manzoor AA, Lindner LH, Landon CD, Park JY, Simnick AJ, Dreher MR, et al. Overcoming limitations in nanoparticle drug delivery: Triggered, intravascular release to improve drug penetration into tumors. Cancer Research. 2012;**72**(21):5566-5575

[56] Costa M, Horrillo R, Ortiz AM, Pérez A, Mestre A, Ruiz A, et al. Increased albumin oxidation in cerebrospinal fluid and plasma from Alzheimer's disease patients. Journal of Alzheimer's Disease. 2018;**63**(4):1395-1404

[57] Miele E, Spinelli GP, Miele E, Tomao F, Tomao S. Albumin-bound formulation of paclitaxel (Abraxane® ABI-007) in the treatment of breast cancer. International Journal of Nanomedicine. 2009;**4**:99-105

[58] Adick A, Hoheisel W, Schneid S, Mulac D, Azhdari S, Langer K. Challenges of nanoparticle albumin bound (nab™) technology: Comparative study of Abraxane® with a newly developed albumin-stabilized itraconazole nanosuspension. European Journal of Pharmaceutics and Biopharmaceutics. 2023;**193**:129-143

[59] Gradishar WJ. Albumin-bound paclitaxel: A next-generation taxane.

Expert Opinion on Pharmacotherapy. 2006;7(8):1041-1053

[60] Ibrahim N, Ibrahim H, Dormoi J, Briolant S, Pradines B, Moreno A, et al. Albumin-bound nanoparticles of practically water-insoluble antimalarial lead greatly enhance its efficacy. International Journal of Pharmaceutics. 2014;**464**(1-2):214-224

[61] Mann JE. Sirolimus protein-bound particles (Fyarro™). Oncology Times. 2022;**44**(14):13-19

[62] He XM, Carter DC. Atomic structure and chemistry of human serum albumin. Nature. 1992;**358**:209. DOI: 10.1038/358209a0

[63] Ghuman J, Zunszain PA, Petitpas I, Bhattacharya AA, Otagiri M, Curry S. Structural basis of the drug-binding specificity of human serum albumin. Journal of Molecular Biology. 2005;**353**(1):38-52

[64] Merlot AM, Kalinowski DS, Richardson DR. Unraveling the mysteries of serum albumin—More than just a serum protein. Frontiers in Physiology. 2014;**5**:299

[65] Fang J, Islam W, Maeda H. Exploiting the dynamics of the EPR effect and strategies to improve the therapeutic effects of nanomedicines by using EPR effect enhancers. Advanced Drug Delivery Reviews. 2020;**157**:142-160

[66] Kiarashi M, Yasamineh S. Albumin nanoparticles are a promising drug delivery system in dentistry. Biomedical Engineering Online. 2024;**23**(1):122

[67] Fu Q, Sun J, Zhang W, Sui X, Yan Z, He Z. Nanoparticle albumin-bound (NAB) technology is a promising method for anti-cancer drug delivery. Recent Patents on Anti-Cancer Drug Discovery. 2009;**4**(3):262-272

[68] Yardley DA. Nab-paclitaxel mechanisms of action and delivery. Journal of Controlled Release. 2013;**170**(3):365-372

[69] Yamamoto Y, Kawano I, Iwase H. Nab-paclitaxel for the treatment of breast cancer: Efficacy, safety, and approval. Oncotargets and Therapy. 2011;**4**:123-136

[70] Belinskaia DA, Voronina PA, Shmurak VI, Jenkins RO, Goncharov NV. Serum albumin in health and disease: Esterase, antioxidant, transporting and signaling properties. International Journal of Molecular Sciences. 2021;**22**(19):10318

[71] Su T, Yang H, Fan Q, Jia D, Tao Z, Wan L, et al. Enhancing the circulating half-life and the antitumor effects of a tumor-selective cytotoxic peptide by exploiting endogenous serum albumin as a drug carrier. International Journal of Pharmaceutics. 2016;**499**(1):195-204. Available from: https://www.sciencedirect.com/science/article/pii/S0378517315304695

[72] Teesalu T, Sugahara KN, Ruoslahti E. Tumor-penetrating peptides. Frontiers in Oncology. 2013;**3**:216

[73] Zheng A, Ning Z, Wang X, Li Z, Sun Y, Wu M, et al. Human serum albumin as the carrier to fabricate STING-activating peptide nanovaccine for antitumor immunotherapy. Materials Today Bio. 2024;**25**:100955

[74] Ma Y, Fang S, Zhao S, Wang X, Wang D, Ma M, et al. A recombinant slow-release PACAP-derived peptide alleviates diabetes by promoting both insulin secretion and actions. Biomaterials. 2015;**51**:80-90

[75] Tseng SH, Cheng MA, Farmer E, Ferrall L, Kung YJ, Lam B, et al. Albumin and interferon-β fusion protein serves as an effective vaccine

adjuvant to enhance antigen-specific CD8+ T cell-mediated antitumor immunity. Journal for Immunotherapy of Cancer. 2022;**10**(4):e004342

[76] Yang YD, Lu N, Tian R. Serum albumin acted as an effective carrier to improve the stability of bioactive flavonoid. Amino Acids. 2023;**55**(12):1879-1890

[77] Shirata C, Kaneko J, Inagaki Y, Kokudo T, Sato M, Kiritani S, et al. Near-infrared photothermal/photodynamic therapy with indocyanine green induces apoptosis of hepatocellular carcinoma cells through oxidative stress. Scientific Reports. 2017;**7**(1):13958

[78] Tomkin GH. Albiglutide, an albumin-based fusion of glucagon-like peptide 1 for the potential treatment of type 2 diabetes. Current Opinion in Molecular Therapeutics. 2009;**11**(5):579-588

[79] Elsadek B, Kratz F. Impact of albumin on drug delivery—New applications on the horizon. Journal of Controlled Release. 2012;**157**(1):4-28

[80] Shechter Y, Mironchik M, Rubinraut S, Saul A, Tsubery H, Fridkin M. Albumin–insulin conjugate releasing insulin slowly under physiological conditions: A new concept for long-acting insulin. Bioconjugate Chemistry. 2005;**16**(4):913-920

[81] Lomis N, Westfall S, Shum-Tim D, Prakash S. Synthesis and characterization of peptide conjugated human serum albumin nanoparticles for targeted cardiac uptake and drug delivery. PLoS One. 2021;**16**(9):e0254305

[82] Abraham MK, Jost E, Hohmann JD, Searle AK, Bongcaron V, Song Y, et al. A recombinant fusion construct between human serum albumin and NTPDase CD39 allows anti-inflammatory and anti-thrombotic coating of medical devices. Pharmaceutics. 2021;**13**(9):1504

[83] Keam SJ. Ozoralizumab: First approval. Drugs. 2023;**83**(1):87-92

[84] Chuang YM, He L, Pinn ML, Tsai YC, Cheng MA, Farmer E, et al. Albumin fusion with granulocyte-macrophage colony-stimulating factor acts as an immunotherapy against chronic tuberculosis. Cellular & Molecular Immunology. 2021;**18**(10):2393-2401

[85] Yang B, Kwon I. Thermostable and long-circulating albumin-conjugated Arthrobacter globiformis urate oxidase. Pharmaceutics. 2021;**13**(8):1298

[86] Wang Y, Han Q, Zhang S, Xing X, Sun X. New perspective on the immunomodulatory activity of ginsenosides: Focus on effective therapies for post-COVID-19. Biomedicine & Pharmacotherapy. 2023;**165**:115154

[87] Maurya P, Singh S, Mishra N, Pal R, Singh N, Parashar P, et al. Albumin-based nanomaterials in drug delivery and biomedical applications. In: Biopolymer-Based Nanomaterials in Drug Delivery and Biomedical Applications. Boston, MA: Elsevier, Academic Press; 2021. pp. 465-496

[88] Karimi M, Bahrami S, Ravari SB, Zangabad PS, Mirshekari H, Bozorgomid M, et al. Albumin nanostructures as advanced drug delivery systems. Expert Opinion on Drug Delivery. 2016;**13**(11):1609-1623

[89] An FF, Zhang XH. Strategies for preparing albumin-based nanoparticles for multifunctional bioimaging and drug delivery. Theranostics. 2017;**7**(15):3667

[90] Li F, Yeh S, Shi Q, Wang P, Wu H, Xin J. A novel thermal-driven

self-assembly method to prepare albumin nanoparticles: Formation kinetics, degradation behavior and formation mechanism. AAPS PharmSciTech. 2022;**23**(7):250

[91] Chali SP, Westmeier J, Krebs F, Jiang S, Neesen FP, Uncuer D, et al. Albumin nanocapsules and nanocrystals for efficient intracellular drug release. Nanoscale Horizons. 2024;**9**(11):1978-1989

[92] Shrestha S, Shrestha A, Kim J, Thapa RK, Kim JO. Recent advances in albumin nanoparticle-based cancer therapies. Journal of Pharmaceutical Investigation. 2025;**55**(1):1-14

[93] Xu L, He XY, Liu BY, Xu C, Ai SL, Zhuo RX, et al. Aptamer-functionalized albumin-based nanoparticles for targeted drug delivery. Colloids and Surfaces B: Biointerfaces. 2018;**171**:24-30

[94] Jahanban-Esfahlan A, Dastmalchi S, Davaran S. A simple improved desolvation method for the rapid preparation of albumin nanoparticles. International Journal of Biological Macromolecules. 2016;**91**:703-709

[95] Shulmeyster GA, Chekmeneva YD, Baibakova MA, Korolev DV. Synthesis of albumin nanoparticles with immobilized and incorporated fluorophores and drugs, properties and release profiles. Nanobiotechnology Reports. 2024;**19**(2):305-310

[96] Srivastava A, Prajapati A. Albumin and functionalized albumin nanoparticles: Production strategies, characterization, and target indications. Asian Biomedicine. 2020;**14**:217-242

[97] Lee ES, Youn YS. Albumin-based potential drugs: Focus on half-life extension and nanoparticle preparation. Journal of Pharmaceutical Investigation. 2016;**46**:305-315

[98] Hosseinifar N, Sharif AAM, Goodarzi N, Amini M, Dinarvand R. Preparation of human serum albumin nanoparticles using a chemometric technique. Journal of Nanostructure in Chemistry. 2017;7:327-335

[99] Zhang K, Han Z, Chen D, Zhang C, Zhang Q, Cai B, et al. Formulating spray-dried albumin-modified lipid nanoparticles encapsulating acyclovir for enhanced pulmonary drug delivery. Frontiers in Bioscience-Landmark. 2024;**29**(10):363

[100] Strojewski D, Krupa A. Spray drying and nano spray drying as manufacturing methods of drug-loaded polymeric particles. Polymers in Medicine. 2022;**52**(2):101-111

[101] Sristi, Fatima M, Sheikh A, Almalki W, Talegaonkar S, Dubey S, et al. Recent advancement on albumin nanoparticles in treating lung carcinoma. Journal of Drug Targeting. 2023;**31**:1-24

[102] Jadhav K, Kole E, Abhang A, Rojekar S, Sugandhi V, Verma R, et al. Revealing the potential of nano spray drying for effective delivery of pharmaceuticals and biologicals. Drying Technology. 2024;**43**(1-2):90-113

[103] Wilson B, Lavanya Y, Priyadarshini SRB, Ramasamy M, Jenita JL. Albumin nanoparticles for the delivery of gabapentin: Preparation, characterization and pharmacodynamic studies. International Journal of Pharmaceutics. 2014;**473**(1-2):73-79

[104] Karami E, Behdani M, Kazemi-Lomedasht F. Albumin nanoparticles as nanocarriers for drug delivery: Focusing on antibody and nanobody delivery and albumin-based drugs. Journal of

Drug Delivery Science and Technology. 2020;**55**:101471

[105] Kundu S, Banerjee C, Sarkar N. Inhibiting the fibrillation of serum albumin proteins in the presence of surface active ionic liquids (SAILs) at low pH: Spectroscopic and microscopic study. The Journal of Physical Chemistry B. 2017;**121**(32):7550-7560

[106] Kianfar E. Protein nanoparticles in drug delivery: Animal protein, plant proteins and protein cages, albumin nanoparticles. Journal of Nanobiotechnology. 2021;**19**(1):159

[107] Tarhini M, Benlyamani I, Hamdani S, Agusti G, Fessi H, Greige-Gerges H, et al. Protein-based nanoparticle preparation via nanoprecipitation method. Materials. 2018;**11**(3):394

[108] Li HY, Zhang F. Preparation of nanoparticles by spray-drying and their use for efficient pulmonary drug delivery. Nanoparticles in Biology and Medicine: Methods and Protocols. 2012;**906**:123-136

[109] Gunjkar S, Gupta U, Nair R, Paul P, Aalhate M, Mahajan S, et al. The neoteric paradigm of biomolecule-functionalized albumin-based targeted cancer therapeutics. AAPS PharmSciTech. 2024;**25**(8):265

[110] Korolev D, Shumilo M, Shulmeyster G, Krutikov A, Golovkin A, Mishanin A, et al. Hemolytic activity, cytotoxicity, and antimicrobial effects of human albumin-and polysorbate-80-coated silver nanoparticles. Nanomaterials. 2021;**11**(6):1484

[111] Yuan Y, Gao H, Jiang S, You Q, Zhou J, Chen J. Magnetic resonance imaging contrast agents based on albumin nanoparticles. Biomaterials Science. 2024;**13**:408-421

[112] Bernardim B, Conde J, Hakala T, Becher JB, Canzano M, Vasco AV, et al. Cathepsin B processing is required for the in vivo efficacy of albumin–drug conjugates. Bioconjugate Chemistry. 2024;**35**(2):132-139

[113] Li J, Zhang X, Pan L, Lin X, Zhang B, Ren J, et al. Combinational strategy using albumin-based nanoparticles to enable synergetic anti-rheumatic efficacy and reduced hepatotoxicity. International Journal of Pharmaceutics. 2024;**656**:124111

[114] Masoumi S, Aleyasin SA, Faghihi S. Albumin nanoparticles-mediated doxorubicin delivery enhances the anti-tumor efficiency in ovarian cancer cells through controlled release. Naunyn-Schmiedeberg's Archives of Pharmacology. 2025;**398**(6):6885-6900

[115] Schmid B, Warnecke A, Fichtner I, Jung M, Kratz F. Development of albumin-binding camptothecin prodrugs using a peptide positional scanning library. Bioconjugate Chemistry. 2007;**18**(6):1786-1799

[116] Cho H, Jeon SI, Ahn CH, Shim MK, Kim K. Emerging albumin-binding anticancer drugs for tumor-targeted drug delivery: Current understandings and clinical translation. Pharmaceutics. 2022;**14**(4):728

[117] Hoogenboezem EN, Patel SS, Lo JH, Cavnar AB, Babb LM, Francini N, et al. Structural optimization of siRNA conjugates for albumin binding achieves effective MCL1-directed cancer therapy. Nature Communications. 2024;**15**(1):1581

[118] Zaleski M, Chase L, Hood E, Wang Z, Nong J, Espy C, et al.

Conjugation chemistry markedly impacts toxicity and biodistribution of targeted nanoparticles, mediated by complement activation. Advanced Materials. 2024;**37**:2409945

[119] Yang B, Shan C, Song X, Lv X, Long Y, Zeng D, et al. Development and evaluation of albumin binder-conjugated heterodimeric radiopharmaceuticals targeting integrin αvβ3 and CD13 for cancer therapy. European Journal of Nuclear Medicine and Molecular Imaging. 2024;**51**(11):3334-3345

[120] Daum S, Magnusson J, Pes L, Fernandez J, Chercheja S, Medda F, et al. Development of a novel imaging agent for determining albumin uptake in solid tumors. Nuclear Medicine and Molecular Imaging. 2019;**53**:189-198

[121] Du Y, Xu J, Han T, Jiang Z, Zhang Y, Li J, et al. Albumin-seeking dyes with adjustable assemblies in situ enable programmable imaging windows and targeting tumor imaging. Theranostics. 2024;**14**(7):2675

[122] Chen Q, Wang C, Zhan Z, He W, Cheng Z, Li Y, et al. Near-infrared dye bound albumin with separated imaging and therapy wavelength channels for imaging-guided photothermal therapy. Biomaterials. 2014;**35**(28):8206-8214

[123] Butt A, Bach H. Advancements in nanotechnology for diagnostics: A literature review, part II: Advanced techniques in nuclear and optical imaging. Nanomedicine (London). 2024;**20**:1-24

[124] Ji Q, Zhu H, Qin Y, Zhang R, Wang L, Zhang E, et al. GP60 and SPARC as albumin receptors: Key targeted sites for the delivery of antitumor drugs. Frontiers in Pharmacology. 2024;**15**:1329636

[125] Wang Y, Shi J, Xin M, Kahkoska AR, Wang J, Gu Z. Cell–drug conjugates. Nature Biomedical Engineering. 2024;**8**(11):1347-1365. DOI: 10.1038/s41551-024-01230-6

[126] Frokjaer S, Otzen DE. Protein drug stability: A formulation challenge. Nature Reviews Drug Discovery. 2005;**4**(4):298-306

[127] Gil-Garcia M, Bano-Polo M, Varejao N, Jamroz M, Kuriata A, Díaz-Caballero M, et al. Combining structural aggregation propensity and stability predictions to redesign protein solubility. Molecular Pharmaceutics. 2018;**15**(9):3846-3859

[128] Pandey NK, Ghosh S, Dasgupta S. Fructose restrains fibrillogenesis in human serum albumin. International Journal of Biological Macromolecules. 2013;**61**:424-432

[129] Bag S, Mitra R, DasGupta S, Dasgupta S. Inhibition of human serum albumin fibrillation by two-dimensional nanoparticles. The Journal of Physical Chemistry B. 2017;**121**(22):5474-5482

[130] Sen S, Konar S, Pathak A, Dasgupta S, DasGupta S. Effect of functionalized magnetic $MnFe_2O_4$ nanoparticles on fibrillation of human serum albumin. The Journal of Physical Chemistry B. 2014;**118**(40):11667-11676

[131] Hoogenboezem EN, Duvall CL. Harnessing albumin as a carrier for cancer therapies. Advanced Drug Delivery Reviews. 2018;**130**:73-89

[132] Carter DC, Ho JX. Structure of serum albumin. Advances in Protein Chemistry. 1994;**45**:153-203

[133] Hornok V. Serum albumin nanoparticles: Problems and prospects. Polymers (Basel). 2021;**13**(21):3759

[134] Radomska K, Lebelt L, Wolszczak M. Aggregation of albumins

under reductive radical stress. International Journal of Molecular Sciences. 2024;**25**:9009

[135] Amighi F, Emam-Djomeh Z, Labbafi-Mazraeh-Shahi M. Effect of different cross-linking agents on the preparation of bovine serum albumin nanoparticles. Journal of the Iranian Chemical Society. 2020;**17**(5):1223-1235

[136] Markovsky E, Baabur-Cohen H, Eldar-Boock A, Omer L, Tiram G, Ferber S, et al. Administration, distribution, metabolism and elimination of polymer therapeutics. Journal of Controlled Release. 2012;**161**(2):446-460

[137] Prajapati R, Somoza A. Albumin nanostructures for nucleic acid delivery in cancer: Current trend, emerging issues, and possible solutions. Cancers (Basel). 2021;**13**(14):3454

[138] Kratz F, Müller-Driver R, Hofmann I, Drevs J, Unger C. A novel macromolecular prodrug concept exploiting endogenous serum albumin as a drug carrier for cancer chemotherapy. Journal of Medicinal Chemistry. 2000;**43**(7):1253-1256

[139] Desai N. Challenges in development of nanoparticle-based therapeutics. The AAPS Journal. 2012;**14**(2):282-295

[140] Nakamura K, Kiminami H, Yamashita A, Abe Y, Yoshino K, Suzuki S. Assessment of the effects of sterilization methods on protein drug stability by elucidating decomposition mechanism and material analysis. International Journal of Pharmaceutics. 2015;**484**(1-2):51-56

[141] Ratanji KD, Derrick JP, Dearman RJ, Kimber I. Immunogenicity of therapeutic proteins: Influence of aggregation. Journal of Immunotoxicology. 2014;**11**(2):99-109

[142] Fukuda M, Nagae S, Takarada T, Noda S, Morita SY, Tanaka M. Potential risk factors of protein aggregation in syringe handling during antibody drug dilution for intravenous administration. Journal of Pharmaceutical Sciences. 2025;**114**(3):1625-1638

[143] Torisu T, Maeda A, Ito S, Uchiyama S. Protein aggregation in the frozen state induced by dropping stress. European Journal of Pharmaceutical Sciences. 2025;**205**:106996

[144] Bhattacharya S, Pandey NK, Roy A, Dasgupta S. Effect of (−)-epigallocatechin gallate on the fibrillation of human serum albumin. International Journal of Biological Macromolecules. 2014;**70**:312-319

[145] Maciążek-Jurczyk M, Janas K, Pożycka J, Szkudlarek A, Rogóż W, Owczarzy A, et al. Human serum albumin aggregation/fibrillation and its abilities to drugs binding. Molecules. 2020;**25**(3):618

Chapter 3

Nanoparticle-Loaded *In-Situ* Gels: A Paradigm Shift in Ophthalmic Drug Delivery

Anupriya D'Souza and Raghuvir Pissurlenkar

Abstract

Ophthalmic drug delivery is inherently challenging due to rapid precorneal elimination, poor bioavailability, and frequent dosing requirements. This research focuses on the design and optimization of nanoparticle-loaded *in-situ* gel formulations for the sustained and enhanced ocular delivery of flurbiprofen. An experiment design was employed to optimize distinct formulations systematically. Nanoparticles were developed using an optimized method to achieve desirable particle size, polydispersity index, zeta potential, and encapsulation efficiency ensuring optimal drug entrapment and stability. These nanoparticles were incorporated into pH-sensitive *in-situ* gel matrices that transition from a solution to a gel upon ocular administration, prolonging retention time and enhancing drug absorption. *Ex-vivo* corneal permeation studies demonstrated a significant improvement in drug permeation compared to conventional formulations. Additionally, histopathological, microscopical, isotonicity, and sterility evaluations confirmed the biocompatibility and ocular safety of the developed systems. The formulations exhibited sustained drug release profiles, reducing the need for frequent administration and improving therapeutic efficacy. The findings of this study establish nanoparticle-loaded *in-situ* gels as a promising platform for ophthalmic drug delivery, offering prolonged drug residence time, enhanced bioavailability, and improved patient compliance. This approach presents a potential advancement in non-invasive ocular therapeutics for the treatment of ocular inflammation and allergies.

Keywords: poloxamer-based gels, sustained ocular release, nanoparticle-loaded *in-situ* gels, ophthalmic drug delivery, antisolvent precipitation-ultrasonication

1. Introduction

1.1 Ophthalmic drug delivery

Ocular drug delivery has been a major challenge, especially when the drug has to be delivered to the anterior or posterior segment due to different protective barriers and elimination mechanisms associated with the unique anatomy and physiology of the eye [1]. Conventional ocular drug delivery systems result in poor ocular bioavailability. The eye is a complex and unique part of the human organs. The human eye is anatomically divided into two main segments: the anterior and posterior segments [2]. Ocular diseases are typically associated with one of these segments. For instance, conditions such as conjunctivitis, glaucoma, blepharitis, and cataract primarily affect the anterior segment, whereas diseases like diabetic retinopathy and age-related macular degeneration are linked to the posterior segment [3].

Due to the eye's unique and complex structure, delivering drugs effectively to the targeted site remains one of the most formidable challenges in ophthalmic formulation development [4]. Currently, over 90% of marketed ophthalmic preparations are administered topically, yet they suffer from poor ocular bioavailability. Several physiological and anatomical factors contribute to this limitation, including tear turnover, nasolacrimal drainage, protein binding, systemic absorption, enzymatic degradation, and the presence of multiple penetration barriers such as the corneal barrier (CB), blood-aqueous barrier (BAB), and blood-retinal barrier (BRB) [2].

The main drawback of ocular drug delivery is achieving and retaining an optimal drug concentration in the eye. Several ophthalmic dosage forms, such as ointments, eye drop solutions, gels, and ocular inserts, have been investigated in order to prolong the ocular residence time of drugs after topical application to the eye [3]. These formulations also increase the corneal contact time, but the blurring of vision (daytime use) has resulted in poor patient compliance. Drugs administered systemically for ophthalmic action also exhibit poor bioavailability to the ocular tissue [4].

Flurbiprofen is a propionic acid derivative that is an NSAID with antipyretic and analgesic properties belonging to a BCS class II with excessive permeability and poor water solubility as it possesses poor aqueous [5]. Flurbiprofen is used topically prior to ocular surgery to prevent or reduce intraoperative miosis [5]. Flurbiprofen nanosuspension was prepared to improve solubility and increase the ocular residence time, thus improving absorption and overall bioavailability [6]. They have the potential to solve the problem associated with the delivery of poorly water and lipid-soluble drugs [7].

1.2 Novel drug delivery system

A novel technique that combines innovative development, formulations, new technology, and a novel methodology for delivering pharmaceutical substances in the body as necessary to achieve their targeted pharmacological effects safely can be described as a novel drug delivery system (NDDS) [8]. To minimize drug loss and degradation, reduce adverse side effects, enhance bioavailability, and increase drug accumulation at the targeted site, various advanced drug delivery and targeting systems are currently being developed [9]. The carriers can be designed to slowly degrade and react to stimuli (e.g., pH or temperature-sensitive) [10].

1.2.1 Nanoparticles

The term "nanoparticle" refers to particles with a diameter between 10 and 1000 nm. By modifying their pharmacologic and pharmacokinetic characteristics, they are used as targeted delivery systems for the distribution of small and large compounds. Polymeric materials have been employed extensively to create nanoparticles [11].

1.2.2 Nanosuspension drug delivery systems

Nanosuspension drug delivery systems involve the formulation of poorly water-soluble drugs into nanoscale suspensions to enhance their solubility, stability, and bioavailability [12]. Nanosuspensions are particularly useful for drugs with low solubility, as they improve the dissolution rate and facilitate better absorption, especially for oral and ophthalmic drug delivery [13]. Advantages of nanosuspension drug delivery systems are enhanced solubility, improved bioavailability, targeted delivery, small particle size, stability, improved drug release, uniform dispersion, controlled and sustained release, and improved drug penetration [14].

1.3 *In-situ* gelling system

The term is in-situ (Latin for "on-site" or "in position") that refers to systems or processes that undergo a change at the site of application [15]. Ophthalmic *in-situ* gelation involves the use of sensitive polymers that get altered structurally with specific triggers, viz. small changes in the pH, temperature, or ionic strength in the cul-de-sac [16]. *In-situ* gel-forming systems are liquids during instillation into the cul-de-sac, which subsequently undergoes rapid gelation to form viscoelastic gels triggered by the change in pH, temperature, or the ionic strength in the cul-de-sac, thereby releasing the drug slowly under physiological conditions [17]. The residential time of the gel so formed *in situ* is extended, keeping the drug concentration optimal, leading to a sustained release and enhanced bioavailability [18]. The systemic absorption and dosing frequency is minimized, resulting in improved patient compliance. In the context of drug delivery, *in-situ* gels are liquid formulations that transform into a semi-solid or gel-like structure upon encountering physiological conditions at the site of administration. This transformation is triggered by stimuli such as temperature changes, pH shifts, or ionic interactions [19].

2. Materials and methods

2.1 Materials

This research was conducted with generous gift samples of active ingredients and excipients received from FDC LTD, Verna, Goa, Colorcon Asia Pvt. Ltd., Goa, and Glenmark Pharmaceuticals, Goa, Molychem, Mumbai, Lubrizol Mumbai.

2.2 Design of experiments

A central composite design (CCD) was employed using Design Expert software (version 13, Stat-Ease Inc., Minneapolis, MN, USA) to optimize the formulation by evaluating the effect of polymer concentration and stabilizing agent on the formulation characteristics, including percentage entrapment efficiency, particle size, and in-vitro drug release [20]. A two-factor CCD was applied to investigate the influence of hydroxypropyl methylcellulose (HPMC E50) (factor A) and Poloxamer 188 (factor B) on three critical response variables: particle size (R1), zeta potential (R2), and polydispersity index (R3). A total of 13 experimental runs were generated using CCD, with five center points incorporated to ensure consistency and reproducibility of the model [21].

2.3 Formulation of nanosuspension of flurbiprofen

The nanosuspension was prepared using the antisolvent precipitation-ultrasonication method. A central composite design (CCD) was applied through Design Expert software (version 13) to propose different combinations of HPMC E50 and Poloxamer 188, resulting in the development of 13 batches (F1–F13) [22]. Flurbiprofen was dissolved in methanol (5 mL) along with the required quantity of HPMC E50 to form the organic phase. The inorganic phase was prepared by dissolving Poloxamer 188 in 20 mL of distilled water at room temperature [23].

The organic phase was then slowly added dropwise to the stabilizer solution under continuous stirring using a magnetic stirrer [24]. After stirring for 1 hour, the solution was sonicated using an ultrasonic probe (Cole Parmer, CVO 18) with an 8 mm diameter at 60% intensity for 10 minutes to produce the nanosuspension. To maintain the temperature between 4 and 8°C during sonication, an ice water bath was used. The prepared nanosuspension was stored for 24 hours to allow the solvent to evaporate [25].

2.4 Preparation of flurbiprofen nanosuspension-loaded *in-situ* gel

Six formulations of Carbopol 974P NF were prepared using different grades of HPMC (E15, E50, and K4M). Carbopol 974P NF was dispersed in varying concentrations along with HPMC in HPLC-grade water under continuous stirring until completely dissolved, followed by overnight hydration. An isotonic solution was prepared by incorporating the required amount of boric acid. The flurbiprofen nanosuspension was then added to the hydrated polymeric solution with continuous stirring to ensure a uniform mixture. The final formulation was filtered through a 0.2 μm membrane filter and transferred into 10 mL glass vials sealed with rubber lids.

2.5 Optimization of formulation variables

For the optimization of formulation variables for further analysis, 13 formulations were synthesized into appropriate HPMC E50 and Poloxamer 188 ratios as suggested by the Design Expert software [26].

Software predicted the best formulation, which was chosen as the optimized one and then incorporated into the pH-sensitive Carbopol 934P NF- HPMC *in-situ* gel [22].

3. Characterization of nanosuspension

3.1 Particle size, zeta potential, and polydispersity index (PDI)

Particle size, polydispersity index (PDI), and zeta potential were determined using a dynamic light scattering (DLS) particle size analyzer. The samples were suitably diluted with double-distilled water to achieve an optimal scattering intensity in the range of 200–400 kcps prior to analysis [27].

3.2 HR-transmission electron microscopy

Surface morphological features of the formulated flurbiprofen nanosuspension were identified by HR-TEM (JEOL JEM 2100). The nanosuspension was diluted with deionized water, and a drop of the diluted sample was placed onto a carbon-coated copper grid. The sample was then examined at magnifications ranging from 2000× to 1,500,000× under an accelerating voltage of 200 kV [28].

3.3 Entrapment efficiency

The entrapping efficiency was evaluated by accurately weighing a nanosuspension equivalent to 30 mg of the drug, dissolving it into a 100 ml volumetric flask, and then titrating it. It was then sonicated in an ultrasonic bath for 10 minutes before being filtered through a 0.22 μm diameter membrane filter. Percent trap efficiency was calculated using the following formula [29]:

$$\text{Entrapment Efficiency} = \frac{\text{Experimental drug content}}{\text{Theoretical drug content}} \times 100 \quad (1)$$

3.4 X-ray diffractometry

X-ray diffractometer (Bruker, D8 Advanced TWIN-TWIN, USA) using X-ray diffractogram was determined. The X-ray diffractometer operated in a 2θ configuration with an accelerating voltage of 40 kV. X-ray diffraction (XRD) patterns were recorded to evaluate changes in the crystallinity of the drug encapsulated within the nanosuspension and to identify any shifts or deviations from the characteristic peaks of the pure drug [30].

3.5 Fourier transform infrared spectroscopy (FTIR)

Infrared absorption spectra were obtained by preparing a simple physical mixture of the drug and excipients. This mixture was placed on the device platform and scanned. The spectrum was scanned over the frequency range from 4000 to 400 cm^{-1} to look for incompatibilities and ensure drug entrapment in nanosuspension.

3.6 Scanning electron microscopy (SEM)

The particle size and surface morphology of the nanoparticles were examined using scanning electron microscopy (SEM) (Smart SEM 5.05, Zeiss EVO LS, Jena, Germany) at various magnifications [31]. The sample was mounted on a gold-coated stub, followed by a fixation process, and then scanned at an accelerating voltage of 15 kV to observe individual particles with smooth surface characteristics [32].

4. Characterization of nanosuspension-loaded *in-situ* gel

4.1 Physical appearance

The prepared *in-situ* gel was evaluated for color, clarity, appearance, texture, and homogeneity [31].

4.1.1 Determination of pH and viscosity

The viscosity of the formed *in-situ* gelling system and the formed gel was measured by using a Brookfield viscometer (Brookfield Engineering Laboratories, Inc., USA, DVE) with spindle 62 and 63 at 10, 30, 50 rpm when the gel had stabilized after 30 seconds, and pH of the gel was measured with a pH meter (Genial, Bioera Life sciences India) [27].

4.1.2 Drug content

Evaluation of drug content was done by sampling nanosuspension, followed by dissolving and suitably diluting with methanol, which were further analyzed spectrophotometrically [33].

4.1.3 In-vitro gelation

It was assessed using a glass tube having simulated tear fluid as a gelation solution. Each formulation was transferred in the vial using a micropipette in a 2 ml gelation solution. Gelling capacity was observed by visual monitoring and measuring the time needed for gelation and the time required to dissolve the gel formed [34].

4.1.4 Isotonicity

Isotonicity has to be measured to prevent tissue damage or irritation of the eye. A drop of blood was suitably diluted with the formulation under test using RBC pipette and observed under an optical microscope at 45X magnification [35].

4.1.5 In- vitro drug release

Using a modified Franz diffusion cell, study was conducted. A semi-permeable membrane is used to separate the donor and acceptor compartments. The sample was placed in the donor compartment, while the receptor compartment was filled with 50 mL of phosphate buffer (pH 7.4) separated by a dialysis membrane. The entire assembly was maintained on a magnetic stirrer and continuously stirred for 8 hours to facilitate drug diffusion at 100 rpm and 37 ± 5°C. Collected samples were analyzed spectrophotometrically at 247 nm [36].

4.1.6 Ex-vivo permeation study

Franz diffusion cell was employed for the *ex-vivo* permeation study of the optimized nanosuspension using goat cornea collected from the slaughterhouse. Phosphate buffer pH 7.4 was used as a diffusion medium in the receptor compartment. Aliquots were collected, filtered, and analyzed by a UV visible spectrophotometer [37].

4.1.7 Histopathological study

A pair of eyes of the goat were taken from the slaughterhouse and stored in 7.4 phosphate buffer. One was used as a control. The other eye was treated with 0.03% of the optimized formulation. The excised corneal tissues were fixed in 10% formalin for 24 hours, followed by preparation of transverse sections, which were then stained with an appropriate dye for histopathological evaluation. The sections under the optical microscope were photographed at the original magnification of 40 [38].

4.2 Optical microscopy procedure

Goat eyes were collected from a local slaughterhouse and immediately preserved in freshly prepared 7.4 phosphate buffer solution. The eyes were then exposed to the formulation containing fluorescein dye for 12 hours. Following exposure, the eyes were fixed in formalin, and longitudinal sections (LS) were prepared and mounted on glass slides for further analysis. The fixed sections were subsequently examined using optical microscopy [38].

4.2.1 Stability studies

The optimized formulation was tested for stability for 3 months at a room temperature of 25 ± 2°C [39].

5. Results and discussion

5.1 Design of experiment

The study evaluated particle size, percentage entrapment efficiency, and *in-vitro* drug release. Analysis techniques included ANOVA, normal plots, and model equations. Each response was assigned a contour plot and a three-dimensional surface plot. The optimal formulation was selected based on software predictions in **Table 1**.

The contour plot for response 1, i.e., particle size, is shown in **Figure 1**, which explains that the increase in concentration of polymer, Poloxamer 188, causes a reduction in particle size.

5.1.1 Influence of factors on response 1 (particle size)

The polynomial equation for response 1—particle size in terms of coded factors [40]:

$$\text{Particle size} = +885.56 + 119.60^{*}\text{A} + 627.12^{*}\text{B} \tag{2}$$

The final equation for response 1 in terms of actual factors:

$$\text{Particle size} = -659.14631 + 3.41717 \tag{3}$$

The above equation implies that polymer positively affects the particle size, implying that enhanced polymer quantity causes a reduction in particle size, which is advantageous. It was observed that the polymer and stabilizing agent concentrations had a significant influence on particle size. Specifically, an increase in both polymer and surfactant concentrations in a fixed ratio led to an increase in particle size.

The model F-value of 115.27 indicates that the model is highly significant, with only a 0.01% probability that such a large F-value could arise due to random noise. P-values less than 0.0500 confirm the statistical significance of the corresponding model terms. In this case, factors A and B are significant contributors to the response.

Formulation code (F)	Particle size (nm)	Zeta potential	PDI
F1	55.60	−5.96	0.264
F2	**191.2**	**38.8**	**0.618**
F3	1170	−20.1	1.000
F4	81.71	24.2	0.308
F5	1801	17.5	0.169
F6	72.26	34.0	0.275
F7	927.3	10.7	0.947
F8	4591	42.3	0.559
F9	2736	8.85	1.000
F10	812.2	−1.59	0.303
F11	903.1	−2.62	0.472
F12	1090	−3.51	0.402
F13	1076	1.11	0.303

Bold values indicate the optimized formulation selected for further studies.

Table 1.
Particle size, zeta potential, and polydispersity index of the nanosuspension.

Conversely, P-values greater than 0.1000 suggest that the terms are not significant. The lack of fit F-value of 1.68 indicates that the lack of fit is not significant when compared to the pure error, which is desirable as it suggests a good fit of the model to the experimental data. The contour plot and 3D surface plot corresponding to response 1 are presented in **Figures 1** and **2**, respectively.

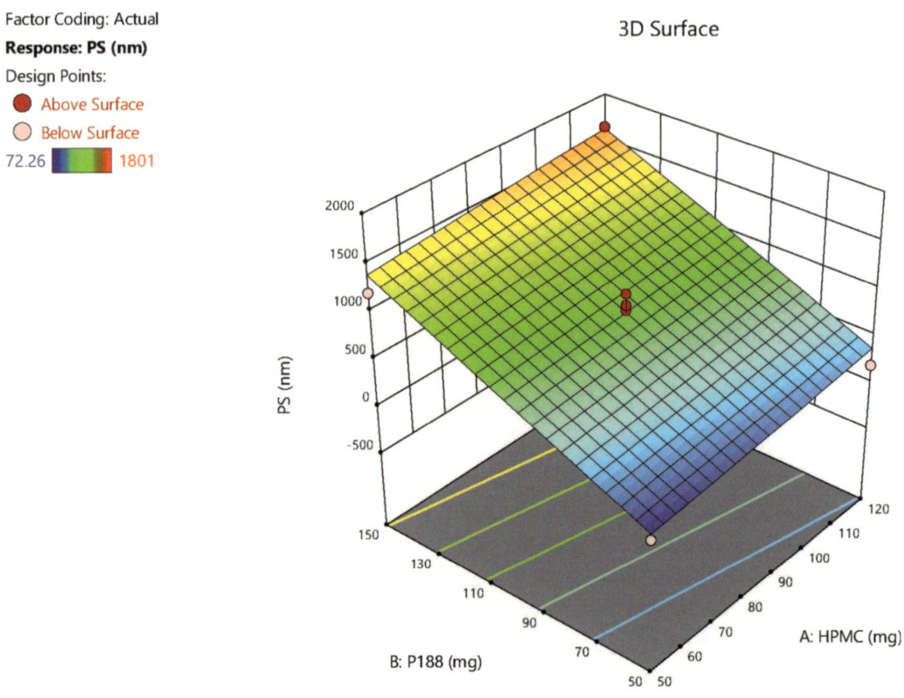

Figure 1.
3D surface plot for response 1—particle size.

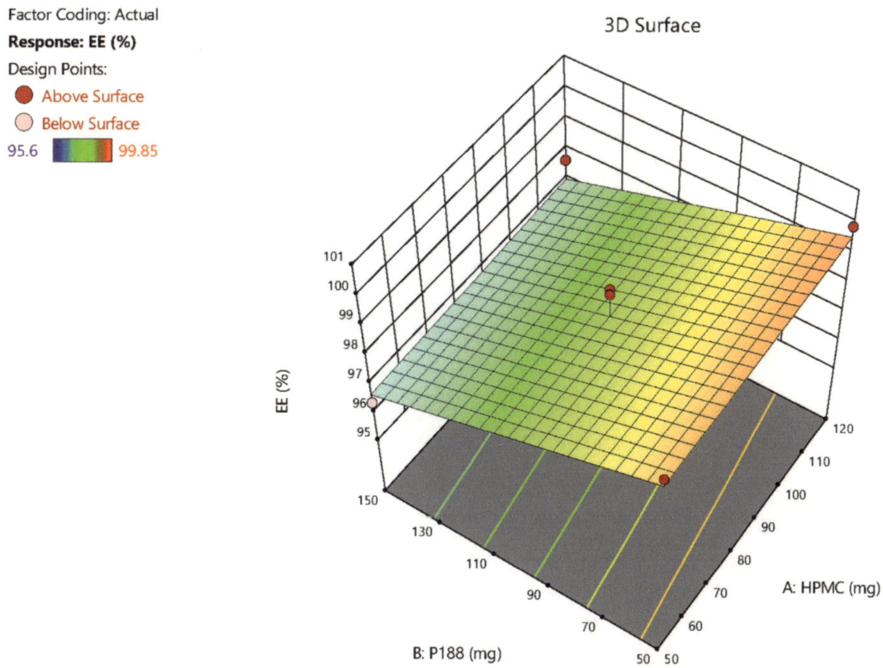

Figure 2.
3D surface plot for response 2—entrapment efficiency.

5.1.2 Influence of factors on response 2 (entrapment efficiency)

The proportion of flurbiprofen trapped in the formed nanosuspension ranges from 95.6 to 99.85%. Thus, it is assumed that the nanosuspension contains the maximum amount of drug. The contour plot for response 2 is shown in **Figure 2**, which shows that the increase in P188 concentration causes a significant increase in drug entrapment efficiency. In the following polynomial equation, the (+) sign indicates a positive effect, while the (−) sign indicates a negative effect on the response. The polynomial equation for response 2—entrapment efficiency in terms of coded factors: Entrapment efficiency = + 98.10 + 0.1651 A- 1.26 B. The final equation for response 1—entrapment efficiency in terms of actual factors:

$$\text{Entrapment efficiency} = +100.22326 + 0.004718(\text{HPMC}) - 0.025249(\text{P188}) \quad (4)$$

Factor A (amount of polymer) has a positive consequential effect on nanosuspension's entrapment efficiency, which is statistically significant, implying that an enhanced polymer mass causes an increase in the formulation's entrapment efficiency, as seen in **Figures 3** and **4** and an overlay plot for experimental design observed in **Figure 5**.

The model F-value of 13.38 indicates that the model is statistically significant. P-values less than 0.0500 suggest that the corresponding model terms have a significant effect on the response. In this case, factor B is identified as a significant model term. When several model terms are found to be insignificant, model reduction can be considered to enhance the model's predictive capability. The lack of fit F-value of

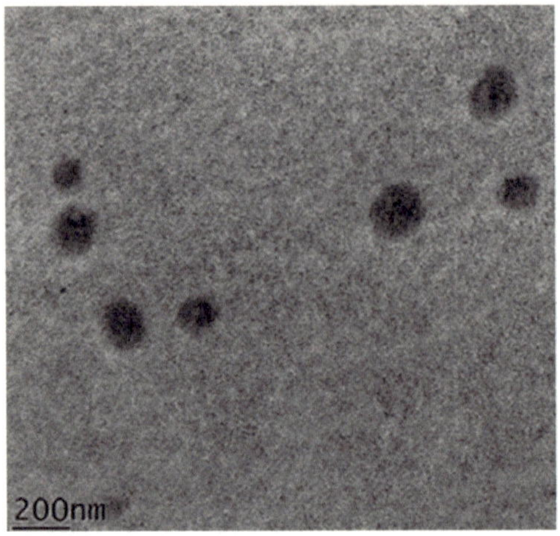

Figure 3.
HR-TEM images of the optimized formulation of flurbiprofen loaded nanosuspension.

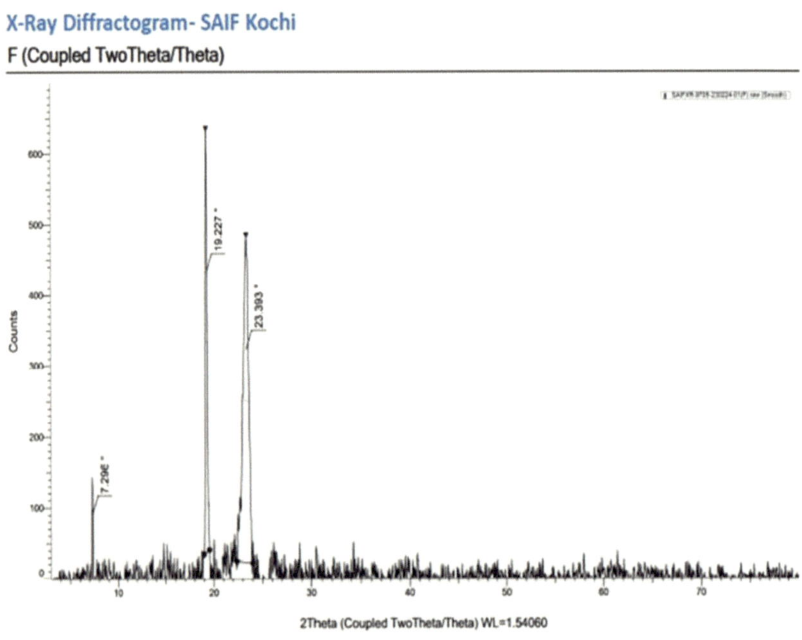

Figure 4.
XRD of optimized flurbiprofen nanosuspension.

1.71 indicates that the lack of fit is not significant relative to the pure error, which is desirable as it confirms that the model adequately fits the experimental data [40].

5.2 Characterization of nanosuspension

5.2.1 Particle size, zeta potential, and polydispersity index (PDI)

The mean particle size for the drug-loaded formulation varied from 55.60 to 1801 nm. The PDI is in the range of 0.169–1.000, indicating that the dispersion is

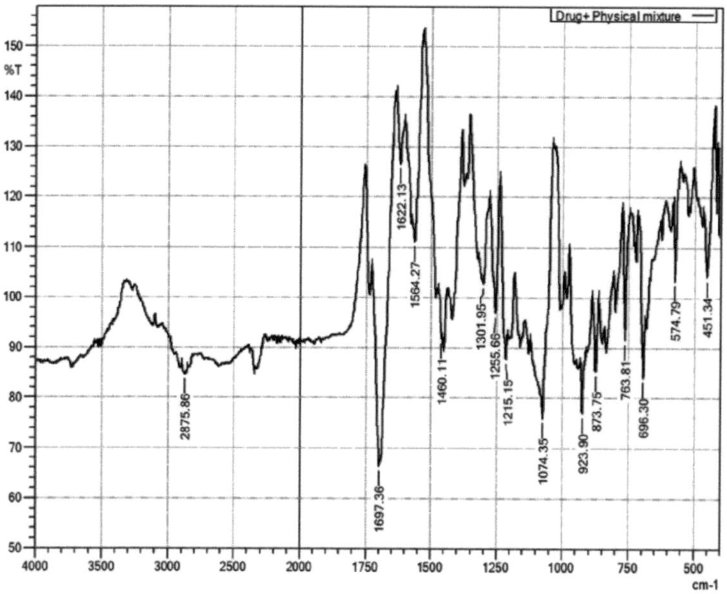

Figure 5.
FTIR of flurbiprofen and excipients physical mixture.

monodisperse. Optimized F2 formulation showed positive zeta potential, and positively charged nanoparticles can aid in successful adherence to the ocular surface and explain significant interaction with the negatively charged mucosa of the conjunctiva and anionic mucin found in the tear film.

5.2.2 High resolution: Transmission electron microscopy of optimized nanosuspension

The morphology of flurbiprofen nanosuspension was studied and shown in **Figure 3**. Microscopic examination of the nanosuspension revealed almost spherical drug nanoparticles with no signs of aggregation.

5.2.3 X-ray diffraction analysis

Figure 4 shows an unprocessed flurbiprofen diffractogram with intense 2θ between 3 and 45°, suggesting its crystalline nature. Flurbiprofen nanosuspension lost its characteristic crystalline peaks, resulting in a halo and dispersed pattern along with a significant broadening of the remaining observed peaks, indicating that the drug's crystallinity was reduced when formulated into nanosuspension. Flurbiprofen nanoparticles' distinctive peak deviates from pure drug spectra, indicating drug encapsulation in the polymeric nanoparticle possessing superior aqueous solubility.

5.2.4 Fourier transform infrared spectroscopy

FTIR of drug-excipient spectra observed in **Figure 5** was compared and analyzed. FTIR analysis validated drug encapsulation in the produced nanosuspension. A significant divergence in the fingerprint region (1400–800 cm^{-1}) was observed,

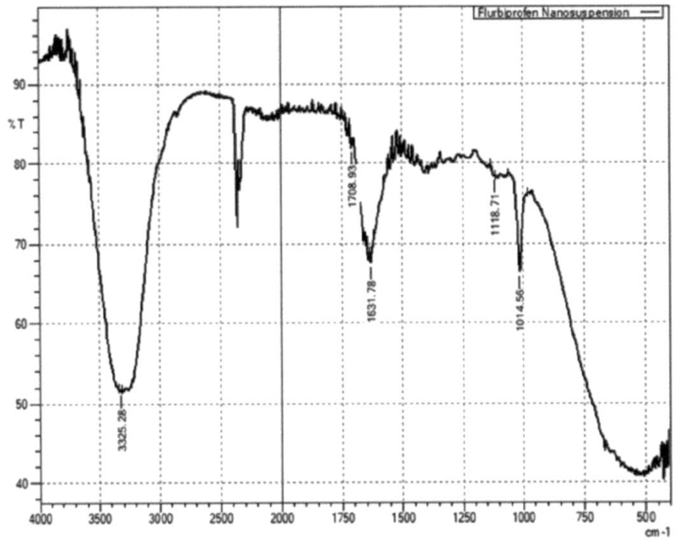

Figure 6.
FTIR of flurbiprofen nanosuspension.

suggesting the formation of new interactions or potential bonding between the drug and the excipients (**Figure 6**).

5.2.5 Scanning electron microscopy (SEM)

As seen in **Figure 7**, the SEM image of the pure drug [A] revealed the presence of drug in the form of irregular shaped crystals indicating the highly crystalline nature of the pure drug flurbiprofen, which owes to its poor aqueous solubility, and [B] shows the SEM image of an optimized nanosuspension which depicted the presence of flurbiprofen dispersed on the carrier surface indicating complex formation suggesting the conversion of flurbiprofen from highly crystalline insoluble form to an amorphous form possessing superior aqueous solubility. This result is in agreement with the XRD pattern of the liquid dispersion of flurbiprofen, confirming the conversion of the crystalline form of the drug to the amorphous form.

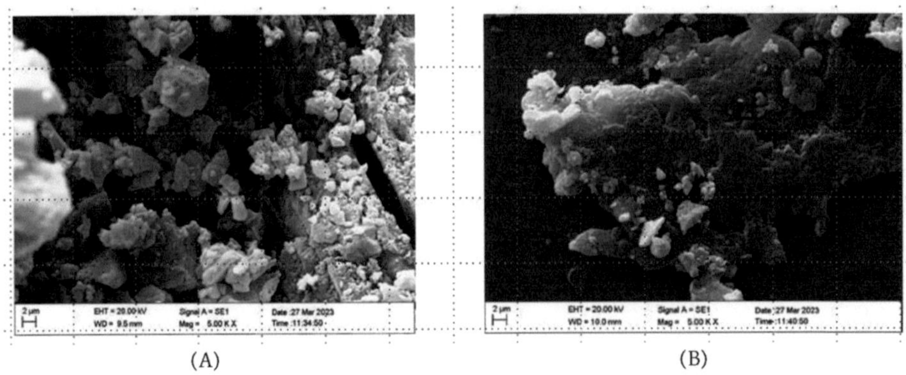

Figure 7.
SEM image of (A) Pure flurbiprofen and (B) Optimized nanosuspension-loaded in-situ *gel formulation.*

5.2.6 In- vitro release study

The *in-vitro* drug release of the marketed formulation showed a more rapid release profile than optimized FB-NS *in-situ* gel. The cumulative release amount from FB-NS *in-situ* gel approached 70.36% at 8 h in a slow and sustained manner, whereas the marketed formulation showed 90% release at 4 h. It was found that *in-situ* gel has better retention of drug nanoparticles and makes this formulation effective in treating. The drug release from *in-situ* gel was fitted to various mathematical model to describe the drug diffusion mechanism. The R^2 value of zero-order kinetic model was close to 1, and the drug release gave a good fit to the zero-order kinetic model suggesting that rate of erosion and subsequent dissolution of polymer gel in a time-dependent manner were responsible for prolongation of drug release. Additionally, when analyzed according to the Hixon–Crowell model, the drug release mechanism from the formulations described changes in the surface area of the gel matrix with progressive dissolution of the matrix as a function of time [40].

5.2.7 Ex-vivo permeation study

Ex-vivo permeation of the optimized formulation of flurbiprofen through the corneal membrane was found to be 94.23% at the end of 8 hours, which indicated good tissue permeability. This provides confirmatory evidence that a significant amount of flurbiprofen from the optimized nanosuspension-loaded *in-situ* gel is permeated through the corneal membrane, which suggests sustained and enhanced release (**Figure 8**).

5.3 Evaluation of gels

5.3.1 Clarity and appearance

The clarity and appearance were evaluated by visual observation against a white and black background. In the liquid form, upon observation, all the formulations were found to be free from any solid foreign particles and opalescent in appearance. Upon gelation, the formulations gave a clear gel with no precipitation or phase separation.

5.3.2 Viscosity and rheology

The dynamic viscosity of formulations F1–F6 was measured against the change of shear rate of gels to investigate the rheology. Upon gelation, the viscosity increased

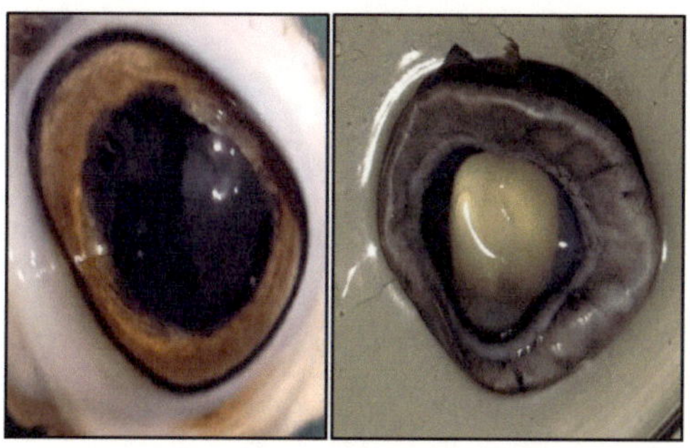

Figure 8.
Appearance of the excised goat eye corneal membrane before and after 8 hours of application of flurbiprofen nanosuspension-loaded in-situ *gel.*

with an increase in polymer concentration. The formulation with 0.8 and 1%w/v Carbopol 974PNF in combination with low viscosity grade HPMC E15 showed low viscosity when compared to HPMC E50, which showed intermediate viscosity. Whereas formulation with HPMC K4M showed high viscosity owing to a higher grade when compared to the latter two. All the formulations exhibited pseudoplastic rheology.

5.3.3 Isotonicity study

All the formulations were evaluated for isotonicity. It was observed that all samples passed the isotonicity test, as no shrinkage or hemolysis (bursting) of red blood cells (RBCs) was observed upon microscopic examination following exposure to the formulations (**Figure 9**).

5.3.4 Sterility test

A total of four test tubes were incubated—two each containing Soybean Casein Digest Medium (SCDM) and Fluid Thioglycollate Medium (FTM). One tube from

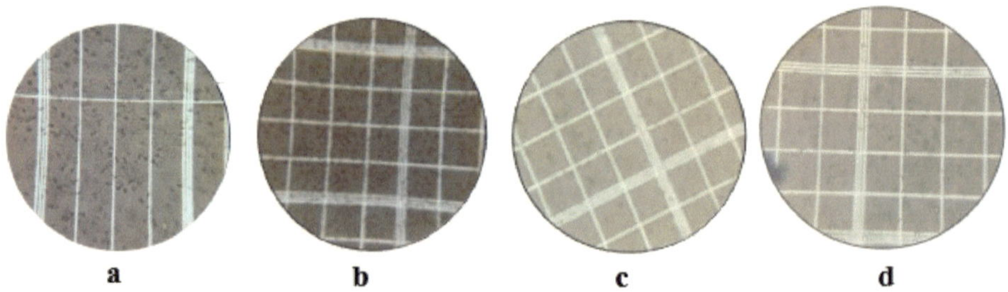

Figure 9.
Isotonicity evaluation of (a) 0.2% NaCl (hypotonic solution), (b) 3% NaCl (hypertonic solution), (c) 0.9% NaCl solution, and (d) FB-NS-loaded in-situ *gel.*

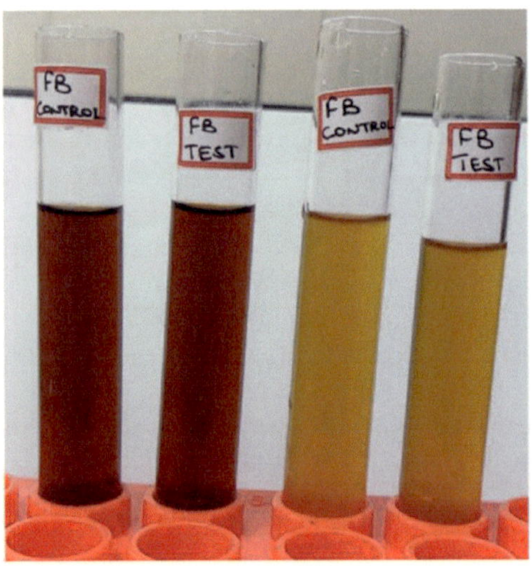

Figure 10.
Results of sterility test on optimized formulation.

each medium contained the test sample, while the corresponding tubes served as controls. After the incubation period, no microbial growth was observed in either the test or control tubes, as shown in **Figure 10**. These results confirm that both samples successfully passed the sterility test.

5.3.5 Histopathological study

A histopathological study of the excised goat cornea was conducted by exposing the eye to the formulation, and no irritation was observed in the image seen through an optical microscope (**Figure 11**).

5.3.6 Optical microscopy

Uneven staining or dark patches indicate damage caused to the corneal tissue. The formulation-loaded cornea had even staining, and no patches were observed. Hence, it is proven to be safe (**Figure 12**).

5.3.7 Short-term stability study

No significant changes were witnessed, and hence, the formulation was considered stable during the testing period.

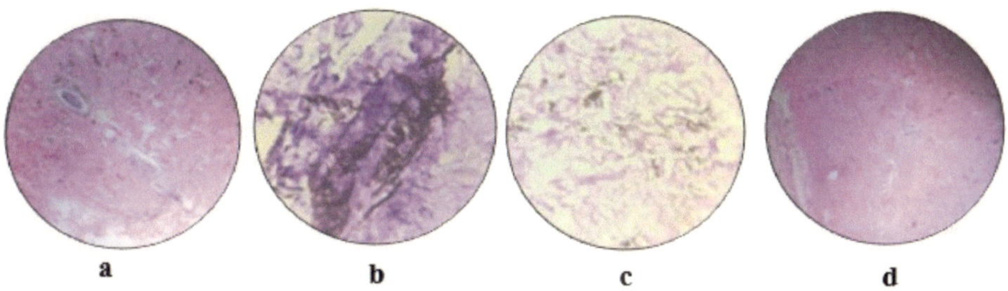

Figure 11.
Histopathology of excised goat cornea (a) Negative control; (b) Positive control—HCl, (c) Positive control—NaOH, (d) FB-NS.

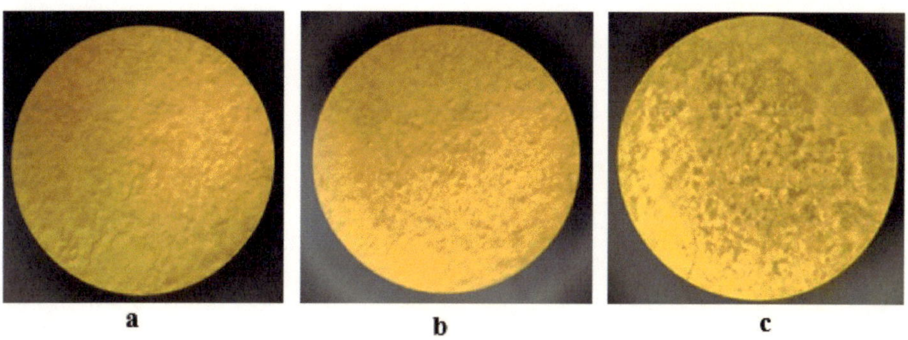

Figure 12.
Optical microscopy of excised goat cornea (a) Negative control, (b) FB-NS, (c) Positive control.

6. Conclusion

Eye drops are commonly used for topical administration due to their ease of use and cost-effectiveness. Effective treatment using ocular delivery of flurbiprofen is a formidable challenge because of poor solubility and short residence time of the corneal barrier, and precorneal variables cause less than 5% of the given drugs to reach the aqueous humor. To address the aforementioned issues, the drug's solubility was improved by creating a nanosuspension and increasing its residence time on the cornea by formulating an *in-situ* gel, which will overcome drawbacks of the conventional dosage form, like rapid nasolachrymal drainage, short contact time onto the corneal surface, etc. Currently, pharmaceutical companies are adjusting their strategies to that of disease management. Novel medication administration has significant benefits, including extended drug action and improved patient compliance by eliminating numerous dosage regimens. Nanotechnology represents an attractive approach for drug delivery. To address these limitations we used two complementary strategies: (1) preparation of a flurbiprofen nanosuspension to improve aqueous solubility and (2) incorporation of that nanosuspension into a pH-sensitive in-situ gel to prolong ocular residence time and provide sustained release. This formulation offers a possible alternative to traditional ophthalmic eye drops by improving bioavailability through the use of *in-situ* gel. Nanosuspensions enhance drug solubility and bioavailability. To extend the ocular residence period of the nanosuspension, it was transformed into an *in-situ* gel. The main advantages of nanosuspensions are their increase in saturation solubility and improvement in the bioavailability of drugs. To further prolong the ocular residence time of the nanosuspension, the nanosuspension was formulated into an *in-situ* gel. The *in-situ* gel-forming technique is patient-friendly due to its ease of administration and progressive breakdown. This formulation aims to reduce dose intake, increase cost-effectiveness and frequency of dosing, and improve therapeutic efficiency. The *in-situ* ocular gelling system is a viable option for treating ocular inflammation, replacing eye drops.

Authors' contribution

Both authors have equally contributed to the design, performance, analysis, and reporting of the research work.

Ethics approval and consent to participate

None.

Human and animal rights

No humans or animals were used in this study.

Author details

Anupriya D'Souza and Raghuvir Pissurlenkar*
Department of Pharmaceutical Chemistry, Goa College of Pharmacy, Panaji, Goa, India

*Address all correspondence to: raghuvir@pissurlenkars.net

References

[1] Al Yabhouni SA, Mozumder MS, Hassan N, Mourad A-HI, Issa MD TMA. Nanocarrier-based, ocular drug delivery: Challenges, prospects, and the therapeutic landscape in the United Arab Emirates. International Journal of Pharmaceutics. 2024;**667**:124899. DOI: 10.1016/j.ijpharm.2024.124899

[2] El-Kamel AH, Ashour AA. Recent strategies for ocular drug delivery: Promises and challenges. In: Advanced Drug Delivery Systems. London: IntechOpen; 2023. DOI: 10.5772/intechopen.106335

[3] Makwana SB, Patel VA, Parmar SJ. Development and characterization of in-situ gel for ophthalmic formulation containing ciprofloxacin hydrochloride. Results in Pharma Sciences. 2016;**6**:1-6. DOI: 10.1016/j.rinphs.2015.06.001

[4] Yang H, Zhao M, Xing D, Zhang J, Fang T, Zhang F, et al. Contact lens as an emerging platform for ophthalmic drug delivery: A systematic review. Asian Journal of Pharmaceutical Sciences. 2023;**18**:100847. DOI: 10.1016/j.ajps.2023.100847

[5] Pignatello R, Bucolo C, Spedalieri G, Maltese A, Puglisi G. Flurbiprofen-loaded acrylate polymer nanosuspensions for ophthalmic application. Biomaterials. 2002;**23**:3247-3255. DOI: 10.1016/S0142-9612(02)00080-7

[6] Oh DH, Din FU, Kim DW, Kim JO, Yong CS, Choi HG. Flurbiprofen-loaded nanoparticles prepared with polyvinylpyrrolidone using Shirasu porous glass membranes and a spray-drying technique: Nano-sized formation and improved bioavailability. Journal of Microencapsulation. 2013;**30**:674-680. DOI: 10.3109/02652048.2013.774447

[7] El Bejjaji S, Ramos-Yacasi G, Suñer-Carbó J, Mallandrich M, Goršek L, Quilchez C, et al. Nanocomposite gels loaded with flurbiprofen: Characterization and skin permeability assessment in different skin species. Gels. 2024;**10**:362. DOI: 10.3390/gels10060362

[8] Huang L, Huang X-H, Yang X, Hu J-Q, Zhu Y-Z, Yan P-Y, et al. Novel nano-drug delivery system for natural products and their application. Pharmacological Research. 2024;**201**:107100. DOI: 10.1016/j.phrs.2024.107100

[9] Adepu S, Ramakrishna S. Controlled drug delivery systems: Current status and future directions. Molecules. 2021;**26**:5905. DOI: 10.3390/molecules26195905

[10] Wang Y, Shim MS, Levinson NS, Sung H, Xia Y. Stimuli-responsive materials for controlled release of theranostic agents. Advanced Functional Materials. 2014;**24**:4206-4220. DOI: 10.1002/adfm.201400279

[11] Patra JK, Das G, Fraceto LF, Campos EVR, Rodriguez-Torres MDP, Acosta-Torres LS, et al. Nano based drug delivery systems: Recent developments and future prospects. Journal of Nanobiotechnology. 2018;**16**:71. DOI: 10.1186/s12951-018-0392-8

[12] Ma Y, Cong Z, Gao P, Wang Y. Nanosuspensions technology as a master key for nature products drug delivery and in vivo fate. European Journal of Pharmaceutical Sciences. 2023;**185**:106425. DOI: 10.1016/j.ejps.2023.106425

[13] Chavhan R. Nanosuspensions: Enhancing drug bioavailability through nanonization. Annales Pharmaceutiques

Françaises. 2025;**83**:251-271. DOI: 10.1016/j.pharma.2024.06.003

[14] Patel V, Agrawal Y. Nanosuspension: An approach to enhance solubility of drugs. Journal of Advanced Pharmaceutical Technology & Research. 2011;**2**:81. DOI: 10.4103/2231-4040.82950

[15] Oishi N, Montes-Moreno S, Feldman AL. In situ neoplasia in lymph node pathology. Seminars in Diagnostic Pathology. 2018;**35**:76-83. DOI: 10.1053/j.semdp.2017.11.001

[16] Rahmi F, Sopyan I. pH triggered in-situ gelling ophthalmic drug delivery system. International Journal of Drug Delivery Technology. 2018;**8**:1-5. DOI: 10.25258/ijddt.v8i01.11900

[17] Kolawole OM, Cook MT. In situ gelling drug delivery systems for topical drug delivery. European Journal of Pharmaceutics and Biopharmaceutics. 2023;**184**:36-49. DOI: 10.1016/j.ejpb.2023.01.007

[18] Ahmed B, Jaiswal S, Naryal S, Shah RM, Alany RG, Kaur IP. In situ gelling systems for ocular drug delivery. Journal of Controlled Release. 2024;**371**:67-84. DOI: 10.1016/j.jconrel.2024.05.031

[19] Vigani B, Rossi S, Sandri G, Bonferoni MC, Caramella CM, Ferrari F. Recent advances in the development of in situ gelling drug delivery systems for non-parenteral administration routes. Pharmaceutics. 2020;**12**:859. DOI: 10.3390/pharmaceutics12090859

[20] Bhattacharya S. Central Composite Design for Response Surface Methodology and its Application in Pharmacy. Response Surface Methodology in Engineering Science. London: IntechOpen; 2021. DOI: 10.5772/intechopen.95835

[21] Yessentayeva NA, Galiyeva AR, Sadyrbekov DT, Daribay AT, Tazhbayev YM. Central composite design for formulation and optimization of rifampicin loaded polylactide-co-glycolide nanoparticles. 2024. DOI: 10.20944/preprints202406.1644.v1

[22] Hassan H, Adam SK, Alias E, Meor Mohd Affandi MMR, Shamsuddin AF, Basir R. Central composite design for formulation and optimization of solid lipid nanoparticles to enhance oral bioavailability of acyclovir. Molecules. 2021;**26**:5432. DOI: 10.3390/molecules26185432

[23] Njoku CN, Otisi SK. Application of central composite design with design expert v13 in process optimization. In: Response Surface Methodology - Research Advances and Applications. London: IntechOpen; 2023. DOI: 10.5772/intechopen.109704

[24] Liu Z, Yang L. Antisolvent precipitation for the preparation of high polymeric procyanidin nanoparticles under ultrasonication and evaluation of their antioxidant activity in vitro. Ultrasonics Sonochemistry. 2018;**43**:208-218. DOI: 10.1016/j.ultsonch.2018.01.019

[25] Jakubowska E, Milanowski B, Lulek J. A systematic approach to the development of cilostazol nanosuspension by Liquid Antisolvent Precipitation (LASP) and its combination with ultrasound. International Journal of Molecular Sciences. 2021;**22**:12406. DOI: 10.3390/ijms222212406

[26] Gonzalez-Mira E, Egea MA, Souto EB, Calpena AC, García ML. Optimizing flurbiprofen-loaded NLC by central composite factorial design for ocular delivery. Nanotechnology. 2011;**22**:045101. DOI: 10.1088/0957-4484/22/4/045101

[27] Udawattha DS, Narayana M, Wijayarathne UPL. Predicting the effective viscosity of nanofluids based on the rheology of suspensions of solid particles. Journal of King Saud University, Science. 2019;**31**:412-426. DOI: 10.1016/j.jksus.2017.09.016

[28] Ibrahim AG, Thomas LM. Formulation and evaluation of bilastine thermosensitive mucoadhesive opthalmic in situ gel. Al-Rafidian Journal of Medical Sciences. 2024;**7**:1-7

[29] Farooqui P, Gude R. Formulation development and optimisation of fast dissolving buccal films loaded glimepiride solid dispersion with enhanced dissolution profile using central composite design. International Journal of Pharmacy and Pharmaceutical Sciences. 2023;**15**:35-54. DOI: 10.22159/ijpps.2023v15i6.47992

[30] Jadhav P, Yadav A. Formulation, optimization, and in vitro evaluation of polymeric nanosuspension of flurbiprofen. Asian Journal of Pharmaceutical and Clinical Research. 2019;**12**:183-191. DOI: 10.22159/ajpcr.2019.v12i11.35670

[31] Tavakoli M, Mahboobian MM, Nouri F, Mohammadi M. Studying the ophthalmic toxicity potential of developed ketoconazole loaded nanoemulsion *in situ gel* formulation for ophthalmic administration. Toxicology Mechanisms and Methods. 2021;**31**:572-580. DOI: 10.1080/15376516.2021.1941461

[32] Aldawsari MF, Moglad EH, Alotaibi HF, Alkahtani HM, Khafagy E-S. Ophthalmic bimatoprost-loaded niosomal in situ gel: Preparation, optimization, and in vivo pharmacodynamics study. Polymers (Basel). 2023;**15**:4336. DOI: 10.3390/polym15214336

[33] Mandpe S, Kole E, Parate V, Chatterjee A, Mujumdar A, Naik J. Design, development, and evaluation of spray dried flurbiprofen loaded sustained release polymeric nanoparticles using QBD approach to manage inflammation. Drying Technology. 2023;**41**:2418-2430. DOI: 10.1080/07373937.2023.2251572

[34] Edsman K, Carlfors J, Petersson R. Rheological evaluation of poloxamer as an in situ gel for ophthalmic use. European Journal of Pharmaceutical Sciences. 1998;**6**:105-112. DOI: 10.1016/S0928-0987(97)00075-4

[35] Gupta S, Kesarla R, Omri A. Formulation strategies to improve the bioavailability of poorly absorbed drugs with special emphasis on self-emulsifying systems. ISRN Pharmaceutics. 2013;**2013**:1-16. DOI: 10.1155/2013/848043

[36] El Sayeh FA, Ibrahim MA, Alqahtani Y, Almomen A, Aleanizy FS. Fluconazole nanoparticles prepared by antisolvent precipitation technique: Physicochemical, in vitro, ex vivo and in vivo ocular evaluation. Saudi Pharmaceutical Journal. 2021;**29**:576-585. DOI: 10.1016/j.jsps.2021.04.018

[37] Alsaidan OA, Zafar A, Yasir M, Alzarea SI, Alqinyah M, Khalid M. Development of ciprofloxacin-loaded bilosomes in-situ gel for ocular delivery: Optimization, in-vitro characterization, ex-vivo permeation, and antimicrobial study. Gels. 2022;**8**:687. DOI: 10.3390/gels8110687

[38] Kesarla R, Tank T, Vora PA, Shah T, Parmar S, Omri A. Preparation and evaluation of nanoparticles loaded ophthalmic *in situ* gel. Drug Delivery. 2016;**23**:2363-2370. DOI: 10.3109/10717544.2014.987333

[39] Ranch KM, Maulvi FA, Naik MJ, Koli AR, Parikh RK, Shah DO.

Optimization of a novel in situ gel for sustained ocular drug delivery using Box-Behnken design: In vitro, ex vivo, in vivo and human studies. International Journal of Pharmaceutics. 2019;**554**:264-275. DOI: 10.1016/j.ijpharm.2018.11.016

[40] D'Souza A, Pissurlenkar RRS. Design and development of nanoparticle-loaded in-situ gel for enhanced and sustained ophthalmic delivery. Drug Delivery Letters. 2024;**15**. DOI: 10.2174/0122103031315270241120053529

Chapter 4

New Potential and Characterization of *Andrographis echioides* L. Ness Stem Extract as an Anti-Arthritic Agent

I. Helen Diana and Vanathi Sundarapandiyan

Abstract

This chapter explored the phytochemical composition and anti-arthritic potential of *Andrographis echioides* stem extract. Qualitative and quantitative analyses revealed a diverse array of phytochemicals, with saponins emerging as the most abundant compound. The extract exhibited concentration-dependent anti-arthritic activity through two primary mechanisms: protein denaturation inhibition and red blood cell membrane stabilization. The extract's effectiveness was comparable to diclofenac sodium, a widely used non-steroidal anti-inflammatory drug. These findings suggest that the phytoconstituents present in the extract significantly contribute to its anti-arthritic properties. The study's results indicate that *Andrographis echioides* stem extract may hold promise as a natural alternative for arthritis treatment.

Keywords: anti-arthritic, phytochemical, secondary metabolites, protein denaturation, cell membrane

1. Introduction

Plants have been used in synthetic drug development and non-pharmacological applications due to their medicinal components. Traditional medicine has used herbal remedies to combat fungal and insect threats since prehistoric times [1]. Despite the widespread use of medicinal plants, their value remains unrecognized in many countries. Phytochemicals, found in plants, play a crucial role in human health by reducing platelet aggregation, activating detoxifying enzymes, exerting antioxidant effects, stimulating the immune system, and demonstrating antibacterial properties [2]. These compounds, including alkaloids, carotenoids, saponins, tannins, phenols, steroids, and flavonoids, have disease prevention capabilities, including antiparasitic, anticancer, antidiabetic, antiaging, antidepressant, and antimicrobial effects [3]. They also contribute to wound healing, accumulate bioactive substances in fruits and vegetables, and enhance stress tolerance [4]. Flavonoids are predominant in plants, with many fruits and vegetables containing anticarcinogenic varieties [5].

Anthocyanins, carotenoids, and lycopene are natural antioxidants found in various fruits and vegetables.

The therapeutic use of natural products, especially those derived from plants, has seen a resurgence in popularity in recent years. These products, depending on their specific attributes, can be categorized as pharmaceuticals, cosmetics, medical devices, nutritional supplements, or traditional foods [6]. Over the past two decades, a significant number of newly approved chemical entities have been small-molecule natural products (SMNPs) or SMNP-based compounds [7]. As a result, governments, international organizations, and businesses are actively exploring medicinal herbs and natural products as a valuable source for new drug compounds. This renewed interest in plant derivatives is partly due to the increased adverse effects associated with conventional medicines. However, plant-based products face several challenges, such as an unpleasant taste and strong odor, which can negatively impact patient compliance. Additionally, their limited solubility, slow dissolution rate, and instability at high pH levels restrict their therapeutic application, often requiring large dosages to achieve the desired effect [8]. Moreover, rapid oxidation and degradation during storage can reduce the concentration of active ingredients in plant derivatives, thereby diminishing their nutritional value.

Rheumatoid arthritis is an inflammation of the joints, primarily caused by a weak autoimmune system and swelling. Symptoms include weight loss, low fever, poor appetite, feeling unwell, and irritation around joints. The disease is not congenital and can be caused by environmental influences or infection [9]. Autoimmune diseases, such as lumps, atherosclerosis, and cancer, can be treated with antioxidants and a healthy diet. Citrus fruits, which contain essential nutrients like carotenoids, selenium, folic acid, potassium, and vitamin C, can also help protect against human malignancies [10]. Arthritis is a chronic condition that causes irregular function, inflammation, and pain. There are 100 types of arthritis, including rheumatoid arthritis, osteoarthritis, and infectious arthritis. Rheumatoid arthritis results from the immune system attacking joints, while osteoarthritis occurs when cartilage becomes tired or less movable [11]. Infectious arthritis is caused by bacteria and viruses, and antibiotics are used to cure it. Synovitis, a type of arthritis, is directly linked to rheumatoid arthritis. Treatment depends on the type and suitability of the individual, with the initial step being a general examination by a doctor. Herbal and nutritional supplements have become important in therapeutic practice and research for rheumatology and orthopedics [12].

Andrographis echioides is an herbaceous plant found in dry areas of southern Asian countries, with a flowering season from March to June and October to December. The plant has elongated leaves with glandular hairs, a slightly quadrangular stem, and a raceme-type inflorescence [13]. The flower's calyx is lanceolate with glandular hairs, and the capsules are ovoid, sparsely hairy, pointed above, and narrowed below. The plant has an average number of capsules per plant and four seeds per capsule. The plant's anatomy includes a well-defined epidermis with epidermal hairs, a well-defined hypodermis, and a chlorenchymatous cortex. The root is composed of a single layer of barrel-shaped epidermal cells, lacking stomata and cuticle, and a compactly arranged parenchymatous cortex [14]. *Andrographis echioides* has been found to have various pharmacological activities. It has been found to have diuretic activity, antimicrobial activity, anthelmintic activity, hepatoprotective and antioxidant effects, anti-inflammatory, analgesic, and antipyretic activity, and anti-ulcer activity. The plant's ethanol extract has shown potential anti-ulcer activity in all tested models [15]. Additionally, the plant's leaves have been subjected to Soxhlet extraction using ethanol as a solvent, showing potential for controlling A. aegypti larvae. These findings suggest that *Andrographis echioides* may be a valuable tool for treating various diseases and infections. Further research is needed to isolate the active principles responsible for these promising properties.

2. Materials and methods

2.1 Plant collection and extraction

This investigation focused on the stem of *Andrographis echioides*, with specimens obtained from Trichy. The collected stems underwent cleaning and shade-drying processes. Subsequently, the dried stems were ground into a powder using a mechanical device and sieved through a 20-mesh screen. A hot percolation technique was employed to extract the ethanolic component from 500 grams of the powdered material. The mixture was maintained at ambient temperature for 24 hours with minimal agitation. Following filtration, the extract was subjected to further analysis at 35°C. Phytochemical screening of the *Andrographis echioides* stem was performed using anhydrous ethanol, chloroform, and aqueous solutions [16].

2.2 Preliminary analysis

Qualitative screening of 18 metabolites was performed using designated solvents to identify the presence of chemical constituents in the root extracts. Quantitative analyses were conducted to evaluate the quantity and concentration of phytonutrients in the extract. These quantitative screenings employed specific methodologies for each bioactive compound, encompassing flavonoids, tannins23, saponins, alkaloids, and phenols [17, 18].

2.3 Preparation of ethanolic extraction

Ethanol extracts were obtained by subjecting 500 g of dried, powdered plant material to continuous extraction with 1 L of ethanol in a Soxhlet apparatus for 10 hours. The resulting extracts underwent filtration using Whatman No. 42 filter paper (125 mm). Subsequently, the filtrate was concentrated and desiccated utilizing a rotary evaporator under reduced pressure conditions. The final dried samples, weighing 50 g, were transferred to labeled sterile containers and stored at a temperature of −20°C [19].

2.4 Protein denaturation model

The control solution was prepared using 1 ml of egg albumin, 2.8 ml of phosphate buffer, and 1000 μg/ml of distilled water and subsequently labeled. *Andrographis echioides* extracts were prepared at various concentrations (100, 200, 300, 400, and 500 μg/ml) and combined with corresponding solvent concentrations (900, 800, 700, 600, and 500 μg/ml), then labeled appropriately. The test solution consisted of 1 ml egg albumin, 2.8 ml phosphate buffer, and ethanol extract at concentrations of 100, 200, 300, 400, and 500 μg/ml.

A single drop of concentrated HCl was introduced to the test solution, which was then incubated at 37°C for 5 minutes. Following incubation, the solution was cooled.

Absorbance measurements for all solutions were obtained using a UV-visible spectrophotometer at 660 nm.

The extent of protein denaturation inhibition was quantified using the following equation:

$$\text{Percentage inhibition} = [VC - Vt / Vc] \text{ x } 100$$

In this formula, Vt denotes the absorbance of the test sample, while Vc represents the absorbance of the control sample [20, 21].

2.5 Anti-arthritic analysis

The Human Red Blood Cells (HRBC) technique was employed to assess in vitro anti-arthritic activity. Blood specimens obtained from healthy volunteers were combined with an equivalent volume of sterilized Alsever's solution. All experimental samples underwent incubation at 37°C for a duration of 30 minutes, followed by centrifugation at 3000 rpm [22, 23].

$$\text{Percentage protection} = 100 - (OD\,\text{sample} / OD\,\text{control}) \times 100$$

3. Results

3.1 Phytochemical analysis

The examination delineates the active biomolecules identified within the stem extract. In light of this finding, the stem of *A. echioides* has been deemed a focal point for the biosynthesis of bioactive compounds. The identified compounds include terpenoids, flavonoids, steroids, alkaloids, saponins, tannins, cardiac glucosides, phlorotannins, proteins, coumarin, emodin, anthraquinone, anthocyanin, carbohydrates, leucoanthocyanin, phenols, alkaloids, and xanthoproteins. Among these constituents, with the exception of leucoanthocyanins and phlobatannins, all others exhibited the anticipated results (**Figure 1**, **Table 1**). The quantitative assessment of flavonoids, tannins, saponins, phenols, alkaloids, and terpenoids indicates potential outcomes. Notably, with the exception of tannins, the remaining phytonutrients, particularly saponins, displayed significant results (**Figure 2**, **Table 2**).

3.2 Protein denaturation model

The results show that *Andrographis echioides* stem extract inhibits protein denaturation in a dose-dependent manner, similar to diclofenac sodium. At 100 µg/mL, the extract (0.37%) is slightly less effective than diclofenac (0.27%), indicating notable anti-inflammatory potential (**Figures 3** and **4**, **Table 3**). The findings suggest that *Andrographis echioides* may serve as a natural anti-arthritic agent, supporting its traditional medicine use.

3.3 Anti-arthritic activity

The HRBC membrane stabilization assay demonstrates a dose-dependent anti-inflammatory effect of *Andrographis echioides*, comparable to diclofenac sodium.

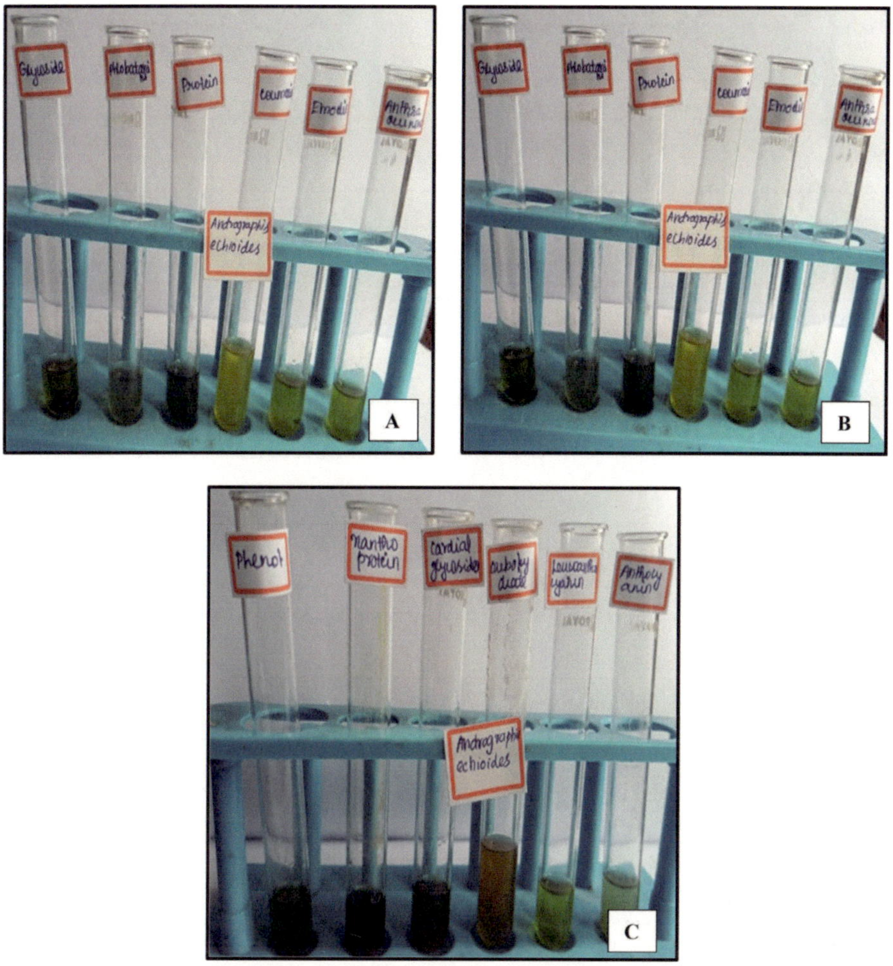

Figure 1.
A, B, and C. Qualitative analysis of ethanolic extract of Andrographis echioides *stem.*

S.No	Phytochemical constituents	*Andrographis echioides*
1	Terpenoids	+++
2	Flavanoids	+++
3	Saponin	+++
4	Tannin	+++
5	Alkaloids	+++
6	Steroids	+++
7	Glycosides	+++
8	Phlobotannins	—
9	Protein	+++
10	Coumarin	+++
11	Emodin	++

S.No	Phytochemical constituents	*Andrographis echioides*
12	Anthroquinone	+++
13	Anthocyanin	+++
14	Carbohydrate	++
15	Leucoanthocyanin	—
16	Cardiac glycosides	+++
17	Xanthoproteins	+++
18	Phenol	++
(+ = slightly present, ++ = moderately present, +++ = strongly present, – = absence)		

Table 1.
Qualitative analysis of the ethanolic extract of Andrographis echioides *stem.*

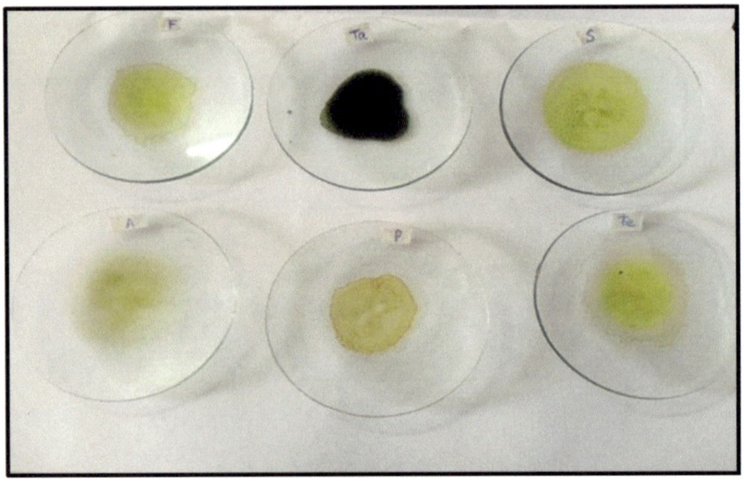

Figure 2.
Quantitative analysis of the ethanolic extract of Andrographis echioides *stem.*

S.No	Phytochemical constituents	Empty Value (mg/g)	Yield value (mg/g)	Final Value (mg/g)
1.	Phenol	18.830	18.846	0.016
2.	Flavonoid	20.656	20.669	0.013
3.	Tannin	20.286	20.326	0.04
4.	Saponin	21.046	21.088	0.42
5.	Alkaloids	19.325	19.595	0.27
6.	Terpenoids	18.771	18.785	0.014

Table 2.
Quantitative analysis of ethanolic extract of Andrographis echioides.

As the concentration increases, the membrane stabilization percentage improves, indicating its ability to prevent hemolysis and protect cell membranes from damage. At 100 μg/mL, the extract shows 0.22% stabilization, while diclofenac sodium exhibits 0.50%, with an overall 81.3% stabilization effect (**Figures 5** and **6**, **Table 4**).

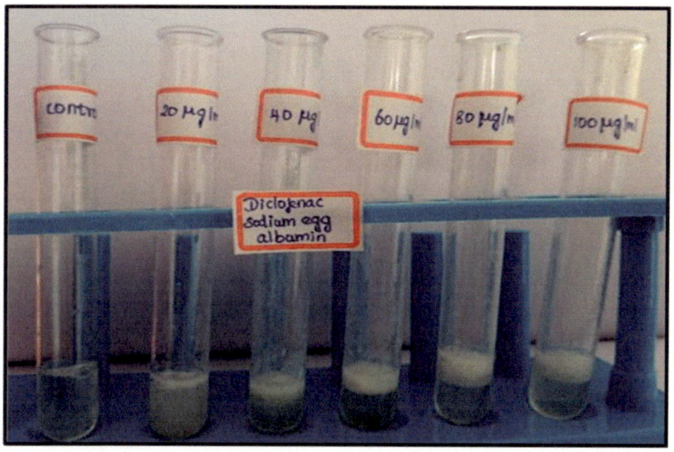

Figure 3.
Protein denaturation assay.

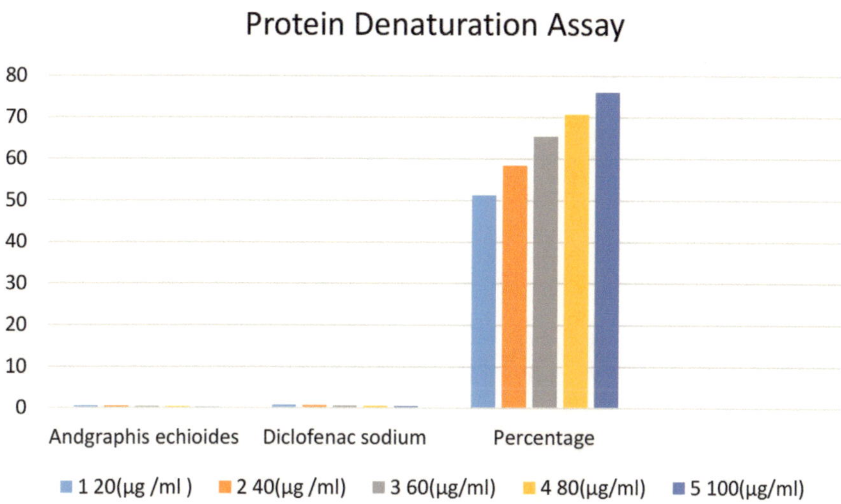

Figure 4.
Graph representation of protein denaturation assay.

S.No	Concentration	Protein denaturation (%)	
		Andrographis echioides	**Diclofenac sodium**
1	20 (μg/ml)	0.68	0.55
2	40 (μg/ml)	0.54	0.47
3	60(μg/ml)	0.50	0.39
4	80 (μg /ml)	0.43	0.33
5	100 (μg /ml)	0.37	0.27

Table 3.
Protein denaturation assay of Andrographis echioides *stem.*

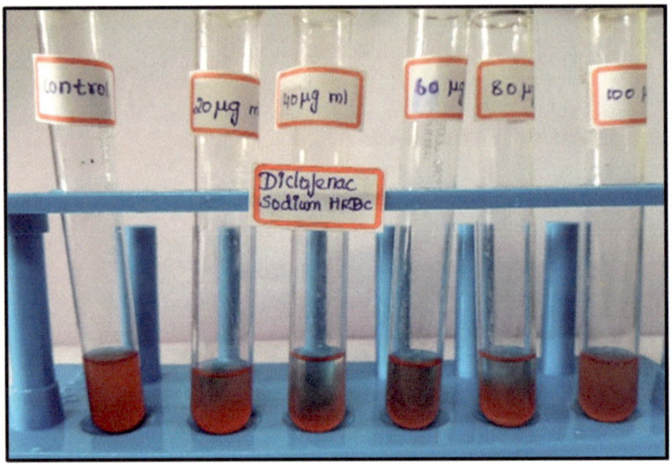

Figure 5.
HRBC membrane stabilization assay.

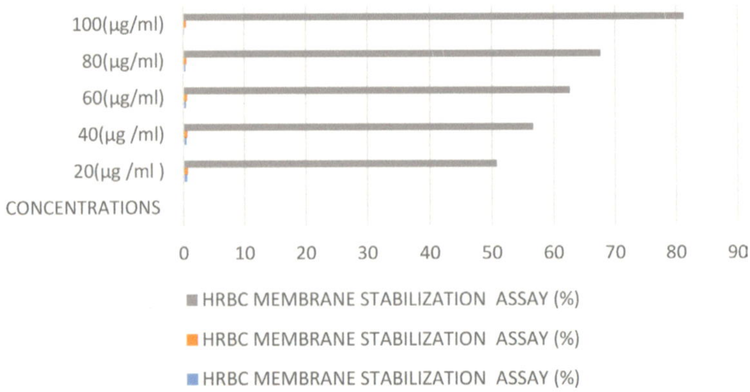

Figure 6.
Graph representation of HRBC membrane stabilization assay.

SI.No	Concentrations	HRBC Membrane Stabilization Assay (%)		
		Andgraphis echioides	**Diclofenac sodium**	**Percentage %**
1	20(µg /ml)	0.58	0.72	50.8%
2	40(µg /ml)	0.51	0.65	56.7%
3	60(µg/ml)	0.44	0.62	62.7%
4	80(µg/ml)	0.38	0.55	67.7%
5	100(µg/ml)	0.22	0.50	81.3%

Table 4.
In vitro anti-arthritic activity of the stem of Andrographis echioides *using HRBC.*

Although slightly less effective than diclofenac, *Andrographis echioides* still exhibits significant anti-arthritic potential, supporting its traditional use in inflammation management and suggesting its role as a natural alternative for arthritis treatment.

4. Discussion

Research conducted by Gurupriya and Cathrine in 2022 revealed that the stem of *Andrographis echoides* contains a variety of biologically active compounds, including steroids, terpenoids, saponins, tannins, alkaloids, and flavonoids. These compounds exhibit efficacy against microorganisms, liver toxins, inflammation, tumors, and free radicals [24]. An investigation focused on the phytochemical composition of Ocimum species ethanolic extract. Their analysis identified the presence of phenols, glycosides, flavonoids, terpenoids, and saponins in the extract [25]. Likely, further studies by Pavithra Kumari corroborated the presence of various phytochemicals in Ocimum species, specifically phenols, flavonoids, saponins, tannins, and alkaloids. Notably, this species exhibited a particularly high concentration of saponins compared to other phytochemicals [26].

A study reported on the quantitative analysis of moisture content, including volatile components, in the tested drug. Their findings emphasized the importance of the final drying process and the rate of moisture removal from secondary metabolites in determining the drug's therapeutic efficacy. Additionally, they highlighted the significance of saponin compounds for isolating diosgenin and their potential in anti-arthritic applications [27].

Barleria lupulina has demonstrated anti-inflammatory activity through the inhibition of protein denaturation. An ethanolic leaf extract of the plant was tested, and the results showed inhibition percentages of 53.78%, 55.25%, and 60.6% at different concentrations in the protein denaturation test. Diclofenac sodium, used as a standard, showed inhibition percentages of 63.3%, 75%, and 79%. The study finally suggested that *B. lupulina* has potential as a remedy for oxidative stress [28].

Another study evaluated the anti-inflammatory activity of ethanol extract and fractions of B. sapida stem bark using in vitro methods, specifically albumin denaturation and membrane stabilization assays. The results showed that the extract and fractions exhibited anti-inflammatory activity by inhibiting heat-induced albumin denaturation and stabilizing red blood cell membranes at concentrations of 200–1000 μg/mL and 50–250 μg/mL, respectively. The ethyl acetate fraction, which had the highest phenolic and flavonoid content, was a key contributor to this activity [29].

The study investigates the anti-inflammatory and anti-arthritic activities of *Martynia annua* ethanolic fruit extract. The extract was extracted using ethanol and phytochemically investigated. The results showed antioxidant activity of 49.1 and anti-hyaluronidase activity of 84.60, indicating its potential for anti-arthritic and anti-inflammatory properties. The extract's potential is significant for treating inflammation and rheumatoid arthritis [30]. Another study assessed the anti-arthritic and anti-inflammatory activities of the methanolic extract of *Peganum harmala* leaves in vitro and in vivo. The extract showed significant antioxidant, anti-inflammatory, and anti-arthritic activities primarily due to alkaloids, flavonoids, and phenols. It also attenuated polyarthritis, weight loss, anemia, and paw edema in polyarthritic rats. The results suggest that *P. harmala* extract has potential therapeutic benefits [31].

5. Summary and conclusion

This investigation demonstrates that the phytochemical screening of the ethanolic extract of *A. echioides* revealed an abundant presence of terpenoids, flavonoids, saponins, tannins, alkaloids, steroids, glycosides, proteins, coumarins, anthraquinones, anthocyanins, cardial glycosides, and xanthoproteins. Phenols, carbohydrates, and emodine were detected in moderate quantities, while phlobatannins and leucoanthocyanins were not observed. Quantitative assessment of the ethanolic extract indicated high saponin content (0.042 mg/g), low tannin levels (0.04 mg/g), and intermediate concentrations of alkaloids (0.27 mg/g), terpenoids (0.014 mg/g), and flavonoids (0.13 mg/g). The ethanolic extract of *A. echioides* demonstrated inhibition of protein (egg albumin) denaturation at concentrations ranging from 20 to 100 μg/ml. Diclofenac sodium, utilized as a reference drug, stabilized the HRBC membrane across the same concentration range. Similarly, the ethanolic stem extract of *A. echioides* exhibited HRBC membrane stabilization at equivalent doses. Both protein denaturation and HRBC membrane assays revealed maximal efficacy for stem extracts and diclofenac sodium at 100 μg/ml. These findings suggest that the phytoconstituents present in the ethanolic stem extract of *A. echioides* contribute to its anti-arthritic activity.

Acknowledgements

I extend my heartfelt thanks to the faculty and staff members of the Department of Botany for providing the necessary facilities and assistance. Finally, I acknowledge all the researchers whose work has contributed to the foundation of this study.

Conflict of interest

The authors declare that they have no conflict of interest or personal relationships that could have appeared to influence the work reported in this paper.

Author details

I. Helen Diana[1*] and Vanathi Sundarapandiyan[2]

1 PG and Research Department of Botany, Holy cross college (Autonomous), Bharathidasan University, Tiruchirappalli, India

2 PG and Research Department of Botany, National college (Autonomous), Bharathidasan University, Tiruchirappalli, India

*Address all correspondence to: helendiana1981@gmail.com

References

[1] Dar RA, Shahnawaz M, Qazi PH. General overview of medicinal plants: A review. The Journal of Phytopharmacology. 2017;**6**(6):349-351. DOI: 10.31254/phyto.2017.6608

[2] Mathivanan D, Suseem SR. Phytochemical and pharmacological review of *Andrographis echiodies*. Journal of Chemical and Pharmaceutical Research. 2015;**7**(7):1167-1171

[3] Saxena M, Saxena J, Nema R, Singh D, Gupta A. Phytochemistry of medicinal plants. Journal of pharmacognosy and phytochemistry. 2013;**1**(6):168-182

[4] Sharma G, Moin S. Medicinal plants: A mini review. Journal of Environmental Science and Technology. 2020;**6**(1):14-18

[5] Ullah N, Zahoor M, Farhat A, Khan FA, Khan S. A review on general introduction to medicinal plants, its phytochemicals and role of heavy metal and inorganic constituents. Life Science Journal. 2014;**11**(7s):520-527

[6] Hoffman FA. Botanicals as "new" drugs: US development. Epilepsy & Behavior. 2015;**52**:338-343

[7] Danishefsky S. On the potential of natural products in the discovery of pharma leads: A case for reassessment. Natural Product Reports. 2010;**27**(8):1114-1116

[8] Lauro MR, Maggi L, Conte U, De Simone F, Aquino RP. Rutin and quercetin gastro-resistant microparticles obtained by spray-drying technique. Journal of Drug Delivery Science and Technology. 2005;**15**(5):363-369

[9] Asuzu-Samuel HO. The prevalence of rheumatoid arthritis on female patients of child-bearing age at University of Port Harcourt Teaching Hospital, Rivers state, Nigeria. GSC Advanced Research and Reviews. 2021;**8**(2):001-007. DOI: 10.5281/zenodo.5195552

[10] Goodman M, Bostick RM, Kucuk O, Jones DP. Clinical trials of antioxidants as cancer prevention agents: Past, present, and future. Free Radical Biology and Medicine. 2011;**51**(5):1068-1084

[11] Scherer HU, Häupl T, Burmester GR. The etiology of rheumatoid arthritis. Journal of Autoimmunity. 2020;**110**:102400

[12] Galatage ST, Hebalkar AS, Gaikwad SS, Kumbhar PS, Patil NN, Desai KD, et al. Rheumatoid Arthritis: Severity Classification, Factors Responsible, Pathophysiology, Current and Herbal Treatment. In: Rheumatoid Arthritis. IntechOpen; 29 Aug 2021

[13] Hossain MS, Urbi Z, Sule A, Rahman KH. *Andrographis paniculata* (Burm. f.) wall. Ex Nees: A review of ethnobotany, phytochemistry, and pharmacology. The Scientific World Journal. 2014;**2014**(1):274905. DOI: 10.1155/2014/274905

[14] Subhashini G, Chitra Devi K, Sundar SK, Rajan S. Pharmacognostic and phytochemical features of *Andrographis echioides* whole plant powder. International Journal of Life Sciences Biotechnology and Pharma Research. 2022;**12**(5):L196-L205. DOI: 10.22376/ijpbs/lpr.2022.12.5. L196-205

[15] Raja RR, Jeevanreddy K. Pharmacognostical phytochemical and anti-ulcer activity of *Andrographis echioides* (Acanthaceae). Journal of

Pharmacognosy and Phytochemistry. 2014;**3**(3):39-49

[16] Diana IH, Sundarapandiyan V. Isolation of novel steroidal Saponin from the stem extract of *Andrographis echioides* L. Nees. International Journal of Environment, Agriculture and Biotechnology. 2024;**9**(6):1505-1516

[17] Nortjie E, Basitere M, Moyo D, Nyamukamba P. Extraction methods, quantitative and qualitative phytochemical screening of medicinal plants for antimicrobial textiles: A review. Plants. 2022;**11**(15):2011. DOI: 10.3390/plants11152011

[18] Velavan S. Phytochemical techniques-a review. World Journal of Science and Research. 2015;**1**(2):80-91

[19] Mathivanan D, Gandhi PR, Mary RR, Suseem SR. Larvicidal and acaricidal efficacy of different solvent extracts of *Andrographis echioides* against blood-sucking parasites. Physiological and Molecular Plant Pathology. 2018;**101**:187-196. DOI: 10.1016/j.pmpp.2017.03.008

[20] Swathi KP, Jayaram S, Sugumar D, Rymbai E. Evaluation of anti-inflammatory and anti-arthritic property of ethanolic extract of Clitoria ternatea. Chinese Herbal Medicines. 2021;**13**(2):243-249. DOI: 10.1016/j.chmed.2020.11.004

[21] Rahmawati R, Widiastuti H, Sulistya E. In vitro anti-inflammatory assay of bitter melon (*Momordica charantia* L.) ethanol extract. Jurnal Fitofarmaka Indonesia. 2020;7(3):1-4. DOI: 10.33096/jffi.v7i3.655

[22] Rahman H, Eswaraiah MC, Dutta AM. In-vitro anti-inflammatory and anti-arthritic activity of Oryza Sativa Var. joha rice (an aromatic indigenous rice of Assam). American-Eurasian Journal of Agricultural & Environmental Sciences. 2015;**15**(1):115-121. DOI: 10.5829/idosi.aejaes.2015.115.121

[23] Farooq S, Shaheen G, Asif HM, Aslam MR, Zahid R, Rajpoot SR, et al. Preliminary phytochemical analysis: In-vitro comparative evaluation of anti-arthritic and anti-inflammatory potential of some traditionally used medicinal plants. Dose-Response. 2022;**20**(1):1-8. DOI: 10.1177/15593258211069720

[24] Gurupriya S, Cathrine DL. Qualitative and quantitative phytochemical analysis of *Andrographis echioides* leaves.(2021). International Journal of Life Sciences Biotechnology and Pharma Research. 2022;**11**(1):148-155. DOI: 10.22376/ijpbs/lpr.2021.11.1.P148-155

[25] Divisha R, Ranganathan V, Vijayakaran K, Elamaran A. Evaluating Ocimum basilicum and Ocimum tenuiflorum leaf extracts for the presence of phenolic compounds. Journal of Pharmacognosy and Phytochemistry. 2018;7(6):2453-2456

[26] Pavithra Kumari HG. Quantitative phytochemical analysis on Ocimum species of Karnataka Ind. Journal of Pure & Applied Biosciences. 2019;7(6):192-202

[27] Chawla A, Singh A, Sharma S, Soni V. Phytochemical screening, development and validation of hplc method for isolated stigmasterol from Ocimum sanctum. World Journal of Advance Healthcare Research. 2019;**3**(6):99-106

[28] Morshed MN, Islam MJ, Shikder MR, Ibnul M, Piash MS, Mostak MS, et al. Phytochemical screening, antioxidant, anthelmintic and protein denaturation activities of Barleria lupulina leaf extract.

Journal of Medicinal Plants Studies. 2024;**12**(3):198-204

[29] Adekola MB, Areola JO, Fagbohun OF, Asaolu FT, Ogundepo GE, Fajobi AO, et al. In-vitro antioxidant and anti-inflammatory activities of ethanol stem-bark extract of Blighia sapida KD Koenig. Journal of Pharmaceutical Analysis. 2022;**12**(2):350-354. DOI: 10.1016/j.jpha.2021.04.002

[30] Kaushik S, Jain P, Satapathy T, Purabiya P, Roy A. Evaluation of anti-arthritic and anti-inflammatory activities of *Martynia annua* L. Ethanolic extract. Clinical Phytoscience. 2021;**7**:1-1. DOI: 10.1186/s40816-021-00250-y

[31] Akhtar MF, Raza SA, Saleem A, Hamid I, Ashraf Baig MM, Sharif A, et al. Appraisal of anti-arthritic and anti-inflammatory potential of folkloric medicinal plant *Peganum harmala*. Endocrine, Metabolic & Immune Disorders-Drug Targets (Formerly Current Drug Targets-Immune, Endocrine & Metabolic Disorders). 2022;**22**(1):49-63. DOI: 10.2174/187153032 1666210208211310

Chapter 5

Applications of Chitosan Microspheres as Drug Delivery Vehicles

Faisal Khan, Aakif Khan, Zia Ur Rahman and Numan Fazal

Abstract

The main goal of pharmacotherapy for any condition is to achieve and maintain the intended curative quantity of the therapeutic agent in the bloodstream or at the desired site during the whole course of treatment. Conventional drug dosage forms frequently cause inescapable changes in drug concentration, which have the negative effects of insufficient or excessive dose, frequent administration, and poor patient adherence. In this regard, various medication delivery and targeting methods are being developed to address these issues and improve overall drug bioavailability. Polymers, micelles, microcapsules, liposomes, and lipoproteins are a few examples of such drug carrier systems. The delivery of drugs is affected differently by each polymer carrier. Typically, synthetic polymers are expensive, persistent, and non-biocompatible. Natural polymers like chitin and chitosan do not present these problems. A naturally occurring polymer called chitosan (CS) is frequently used in medicinal applications because of its affordability, biodegradability, biocompatibility, non-toxic makeup, and capacity to cling to mucosal surfaces. Because of its cationic characteristics, CS can interact with polyanions to produce polyelectrolyte complexes. CS has thus shown to be particularly useful in improving the dissolving of insoluble medicines and in multiparticulate drug delivery. Chitosan has emerged as a prospective natural polymer for the formulation of microspheres and microcapsules. Ionotropic gelation, spray drying, emulsion phase separation, simple coacervation, and complex coacervation are some of the techniques used in chitosan microencapsulation. This chapter will primarily concentrate on the synthesis and characterization of chitosan microspheres, as well as their use in novel drug delivery systems.

Keywords: chitosan, microspheres, nanoparticles, drug delivery, micelles

1. Introduction

Drug delivery seeks to maximize the amount of medications that are available at particular sites in the body for a predetermined amount of time. Reaching the targeted site of action is a common factor that reduces the potency of many medications [1]. In traditional forms of administration, the majority of the medication spreads throughout the body depending on its physicochemical and biochemical properties, with just a tiny percentage of the supplied dose often reaching the target site. Therefore, designing a drug delivery system that maximizes a drug's curative efficacy while reducing its hazardous side effects *in vivo* presents a difficult task. Utilizing colloidal drug carriers, which enable targeted or site-specific drug delivery combined with ideal drug release patterns, is one strategy to overcome this challenge. Paul Ehrlich's idea of minuscule medication-loaded "magic bullets" more than a century ago was the inspiration for the idea of using submicron drug delivery systems for targeted drug delivery. Liposomes and micro/nanoparticles have been widely researched among these carriers. Liposomes do, however, have some technological drawbacks, such as poor repeatability, instability, and ineffective drug entrapment. However, a number of low molecular weight medications on the market now use liposomal technology. Alternative drug carriers that get around many of these problems include polymeric nanoparticles, which are more reproducible and stable than liposomes. The use of nano- and microparticles in the particulate drug delivery system is a physical method of modifying the pharmacokinetic and pharmacodynamic characteristics of active pharmaceutical ingredients (APIs) [2]. Because of their capacity to target certain tissues, get to molecular targets, and regulate medication release, these nanoparticles have attracted a lot of interest in the pharmaceutical industry. Nanoparticles are solid colloidal drug carriers with diameters between 10 and 1000 nm that are constructed from synthetic, natural, or semi-artificial polymers that enclose the drug molecules of interest [3]. Chitosan offers benefits over alternative polymeric carriers for nanoparticulate drug administration due to its biodegradability, biocompatibility, simplicity of formulation, variety in application, and low toxicity [4, 5]. When the active ingredient is dissolved, entrapped, encapsulated, adsorbed, or chemically linked to these nanoparticles, they can be employed therapeutically as vaccine adjuvants or drug carriers. Both synthetic and natural polymers can be utilized to produce nanoparticles. There are two distinct kinds of nanoparticles: nanospheres and nanocapsules, which differ in how they are synthesized [6]. Nanocapsules have a membrane-wall construction that traps pharmaceuticals in the interior or adsorbs them to the outside, while nanospheres have a monolithic structure that disperses or adsorbs drugs onto their surfaces. Due to the difficulty in distinguishing between these particles' matrix and membrane types, the term "nanoparticles" is usually used. In addition to having the ability to deliver drugs via non-invasive channels including the oral, nasal, and ocular routes, nanoparticles have also been shown to be efficient as adjuvants in vaccines. There is currently no perfect nanoparticle system, despite these benefits. Heat, organic solvents, or high shear forces are frequently used to create nanoparticles from water-insoluble polymers, which can compromise the stability of medications. In addition, time and resources are expended in the several processes needed for complicated preparation techniques including solvent evaporation and emulsion polymerization [6, 7]. However, water-soluble polymers offer softer and easier preparation techniques without the requirement for strong shear forces or organic solvents. Chitosan has thus received the most attention among water-soluble polymers because of its advantageous characteristics as a polymeric carrier for nanoparticles, including biocompatibility, biodegradability, non-toxicity, as well as cost-effectiveness. Additionally, chitosan has a positive charge and has actions that improve absorption, making it a desirable substance for drug administration. Chitosan microspheres have undergone substantial development and study for medicinal uses during the past 20 years. Chitosan microspheres are used in drug delivery systems due to their unique features as they allow for controlled drug release, increase the bioavailability of compounds that degrade, and increase membrane permeability. Several studies have been done on the nasal medication delivery of proteins, peptides, and vaccinations using chitosan microspheres [8–10]. Different chemical modifications have been used to increase the bioavailability and membrane permeability of chitosan microspheres and produce sustained drug release. Chitosan can be modified in this way by being thiolated using 2-iminothiolane [11]. Hyaluronan or pluronic F127® have also been added to chitosan microsphere formulations to further enhance their characteristics [12] or pluronic F127® [13]. Through their synergistic impact, the combination of chitosan microspheres and the powerful immunostimulatory adjuvant LTK63 is a successful method for enhancing the potency of nasal vaccines [14]. The techniques used to prepare chitosan microspheres, as well as their uses and method of entry into cells, are the main topics to be discussed in this chapter.

2. Chitosan (CS)

A polysaccharide made of glucosamine and N-acetylglucosamine, chitosan is a naturally occurring substance that is produced by partially deacetylating chitin, the main building block of crab exoskeletons [15]. Chitin from the shells of crabs, shrimp, and krill, which are plentiful waste byproducts of the shellfish processing industry, is deacetylated in order to produce chitosan [16]. The word "chitosan" signifies a variety of polymers with differential molecular masses, viscosities, and levels of deacetylation, pKa values, and other characteristics. One amino group and two hydroxyl groups, which may interact with acidic environments, are present in the chitosan molecule. The removal of the acetate moiety from chitin results in the formation of chitosan, which is thought to be the most significant chitin derivative as depicted in the following **Figure 1**. The pKa value of the amino group in chitosan is roughly 6.5; chitosan thus has a positive charge and is soluble in acidic liquids. This pH and the level of deacetylation effect the size of its charge density. Chitosan's amino group makes it possible for it to interact chemically with anionic systems, thus changing the physicochemical

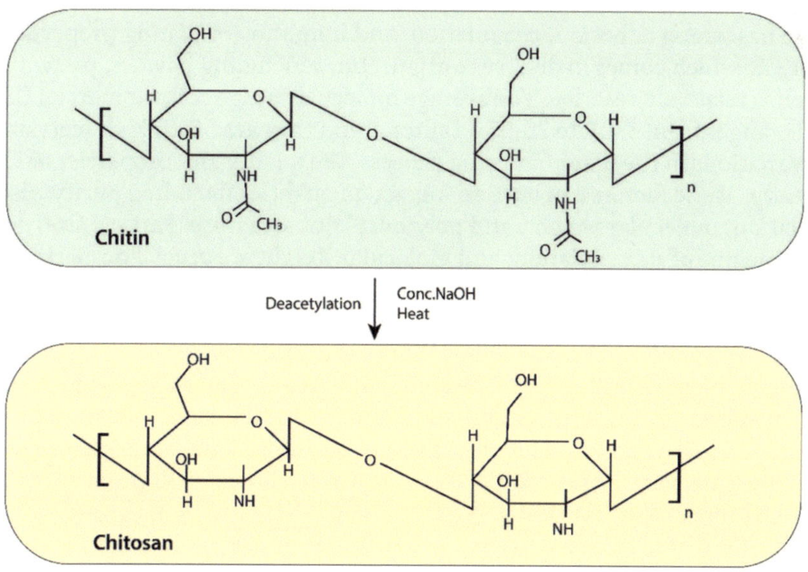

Figure 1.
Deacetylation of chitin to chitosan. Figure was adopted and redesigned from the work of Mohammed et al. [15].

characteristics of these mixtures [15]. Additionally, chitosan's free amino group is easily accessible and exhibits interaction with various anionic polymers.

Chitosan is regarded as a very potential polymer owing to its non-hazardous polycationic, biologically compatible, and biodegradable properties. Its mucoadhesive and permeation-enhancing attributes are especially noteworthy. Chitosan's potent mucoadhesive ability is essential for medication administration through mucosal channels [10, 15]. Chitosan's positive charge also enables it to interact with mucin layers and tight junctions, which opens up the tight junctions of mucosal barriers and promotes the paracellular transit of hydrophilic macromolecules [17, 18]. Chitosan has thus the potential to improve mucosal medication penetration because of its powerful mucoadhesive characteristics. Studies on medication delivery via the nasal and oral routes have demonstrated that co-administration of chitosan with macromolecules considerably increases their ability to pass the mucosal barrier [4, 19]. The improved mucoadhesion between the formulation and the nasal tissues and the temporary action of chitosan on the paracellular pathways have both been demonstrated to contribute to the chitosan's ability to increase absorption. Furthermore, chitosan has been shown by Dodane et al. to alter interstitial permeation [18]. The following sections highlight numerous significant properties of chitosan.

2.1 Properties of chitosan

Due to the existence of free amino groups, the cationic polysaccharide chitosan (CS) is insoluble in water at neutral or basic pH levels. However, the amino groups may undergo protonation in an acidic pH, which causes water solubility. The dissemination of unbound amino and N-acetyl groups affects how soluble CS is. Usually, 1–3% concentrations of aqueous acetic acid are used to dissolve CS [3, 16]. Moreover, CS does not cause allergic reactions or tissue rejection because it is biocompatible with living tissues. It slowly degrades into harmless byproducts (amino sugars) that the body can fully absorb. Furthermore, CS has antibacterial qualities and has the capacity to absorb hazardous metals like lead, cadmium, and mercury.

It also has strong adhesion, coagulation, and immunostimulating properties. The polymer CS, which comes in diverse configurations including powder, paste, film, and fiber, is relatively reactive. The average molecular weight of commercial CS products ranges from 3800 to 20,000 Daltons, and they are 66–95% deacetylated [3]. Due to variations in the manufacturing process, the quality and properties of CS can vary greatly. These factors can have an impact on qualities including purity, viscosity, deacetylation, molecular weight, and polymorphous structure. Particle size, density, viscosity, degree of deacetylation, and molecular weight are crucial properties of medicinal formulations based on CS.

When included in CS formulations, CS also exhibits good bioadhesive properties that lower the rate of medication removal from the nasal cavity and consequently increase drug bioavailability [20]. The ability of CS to chelate allows for the selective binding of substances including cholesterol, lipids, metal ions, proteins, and cancer cells. A good cationic polymer for membrane production is CS. For particular uses, Chitosan polymers can be chemically transformed to change their properties such as solubility, mucoadhesion, and persistence. The $-NH_2$ and $-OH$ groups are the alteration sites that are most active in CS. Modified chitosan polymers are typically created through graft copolymerization, curing, and blending. Graft copolymerization entails the covalent linking of polymers and curing entails the creation of three-dimensional linkages within the polymer mass through thermal, electrochemical, or

UV radiation processing. Blending entails the straightforward mixing of two or more polymers. Physical or chemical methods can be used to make these alterations [20].

2.1.1 Physical modifications

Chitosan can be physically transformed by blending, which entails the amalgamation of several polymers. A simple and affordable method for changing the characteristics of polymers is blending. The characteristics and effectiveness of the mix can be customized to meet particular application needs by varying the ratios of the polymers being combined. When combining various polymers to create desired properties and functionalities, blending enables adaptability. With the use of this method, the properties of chitosan can be improved or changed without the need of significant chemical alterations. To get the intended result, it is crucial to carefully choose compatible polymers and optimize the blending procedure [20].

A promising method for oral medication delivery involves mixing chitosan with hydrophilic polymers like poly(vinyl alcohol), poly(vinyl pyrrolidone), and poly(ethylene oxide). The mechanical qualities, notably the tensile strength, of chitosan films can be improved by adding PVA, PVP, or PEO to them. Additionally, combining chitosan with PVA can enhance the barrier qualities of chitosan films, particularly their water vapor permeability. With the use of this blending process, the positive traits of PVA and the beneficial features of chitosan—such as biocompatibility and mucoadhesive capabilities—are combined to produce improved performance for applications involving oral medication delivery [21]. Chitosan films for controlled drug delivery have increased mechanical qualities (tensile strength), thanks to the chemical affinities between chitosan and PVA [22]. Amoxicillin, which is manufactured using a cross-linked chitosan/PVP blend with glutaraldehyde to generate a semi-interpenetrating polymer (semi-IPN), serves as an illustration of physical alteration in controlled drug delivery [23]. Fourier transform infrared spectroscopy (FTIR) has demonstrated that the protonation of chitosan's amino group results in the formation of the semi-IPN. In addition to FTIR, other techniques for characterizing chitosan blends include differential scanning calorimetry (DSC) [24], X-ray diffraction (XRD) [25], FTIR spectroscopy, and rheology [26], facilitating comprehension of how processing affects bonding and flow qualities.

2.1.2 Chemical modifications

Chemical modification entails modifying a compound's functional groups using a variety of techniques. These techniques include chemical reactions, enzymatic grafting, photochemical modifications, plasma-induced modifications, radiation-induced modifications, and radiation-induced modifications. To acquire desired traits and functions, each approach enables precise modifications to the compound's structure and functional groups [27]. Chemical chitosan modification may result in a number of derivatives like quaternized chitosan, thiolated chitosan, carboxylated chitosan, amphiphilic chitosan, chitosan with chelating agents, PEGylated chitosan, and lactose-modified chitosan. Because chitosan contains primary amine (−NH2) groups, which act as reactive sites for changing its chemical structure, chemical modification thus makes use of these groups. These alterations allow for the creation of chitosan derivatives with a variety of characteristics and functions, making them appropriate for use in a variety of medicinal applications [27], such as reacting them with sulfates, citrates, and phosphates [28], to enhance their stability as well as drug encapsulation efficiency [29]. N-trimethyl chitosan chloride (TMC), a quaternized chitosan, has been created, for instance, to increase the solubility of chitosan in intestinal fluid [30]. The intestinal penetration of hydrophilic macromolecular medicines is thus improved by the two versions of TMC, TMC 40 and TMC 60. By combining NP with chitosan that has been thiolated, the mucoadhesiveness of chitosan is further improved [31]. Trimethyl chitosan (TMC), dimethylethyl chitosan (DMEC), diethylmethyl chitosan (DEMC), and triethyl chitosan (TEC) are only a few of the derivatives that can be produced by quaternizing chitosan. By making tight connections easier to open, chitosan's quaternization increases the permeability of molecules like insulin. This characteristic has been discovered in research utilizing Caco-2 cells, where quaternized chitosan derivatives have exhibited better insulin permeability [32]. Currently, chitosan-thioglycolic acid, chitosan-cysteine, chitosan-glutathione, and chitosan-thioethylamidine are among the thiolated chitosan derivatives used. When compared to TMC nanoparticles, TMC-cysteine-based nanoparticles have shown considerable gains in mucoadhesion and penetration. The addition of cysteine as a thiol group in TMC thus improves the mucoadhesion and penetration capacities of the nanoparticles by strengthening their adhesive qualities to mucosal surfaces [33]. To acquire pH-sensitive characteristics, poly (methyl methacrylate) is grafted with carboxylated chitosan. In simulated stomach fluid and simulated intestinal fluid, the NPs produced with the grafted polymer and insulin showed very limited drug release and instantaneous release, respectively [34]. For their application in the administration of drugs to various parts of the gastrointestinal tract (GIT), d,l-lactic acid and chitosan can be chemically linked to create a pH-sensitive polymer gel [35]. Through polyionic interactions, the lactose alteration of the chitosan backbone (1-deoxylactit-1-yl chitosan) is being used to create colloidal coacervates that are highly uniform and tiny (200 nm) nanoparticles [36, 37]. Chitosan microspheres are synthesized by various techniques. Some of these widely used methods are discussed below.

2.2 Methods of chitosan microsphere preparation

To increase drug bioavailability and control release, particularly for biodegradable compounds like proteins, chitosan microspheres, and nanoparticles are widely used. Additionally, they help hydrophilic molecules pass through epithelial layers more easily. Chitosan molecules are cross-linked during the creation of chitosan microspheres by interactions with particular concentrations of multivalent anions. Depending on the procedures used, the cross-linking process can take place in acidic, neutral, or basic conditions. Chitosan microspheres or nanoparticles can be produced through a variety of techniques, including modified emulsification, ionotropic gelation, glutaraldehyde cross-linking, thermal cross-linking, and precipitation-chemical cross-linking [4, 5]. A number of factors, including the target particle size, the drug's chemical and thermal stability, the reproducibility of release profiles, the stability of the finished product, and any potential toxicity, must be taken into consideration when choosing a specific process for making chitosan microspheres. The type of delivery device being utilized and the makeup of the active drug molecule also significantly influence which approach is the best among the available possibilities [5].

2.2.1 Emulsion cross-linking

In this method, the reactive amine groups of chitosan are used for making chitosan microspheres by a chemical cross-linking process, together with cross-linking chemicals like glutaraldehyde. The process involves the emulsification of an aqueous chitosan solution to make a water-in-oil (w/o) emulsion. A surfactant is used to stabilize the emulsion, and the cross-linking agent is added to make the droplets harder. The resultant microspheres are filtered, and then dried after being rinsed with n-hexane and alcohol. By altering the extent of chemical bonding and the rate of stirring during the process of emulsification, the size of the microspheres may be managed. Despite being often used to create chitosan microspheres, the emulsion cross-linking approach has a number of drawbacks such as the time-consuming process, the use of strong cross-linking chemicals that might interfere with the active drug molecule, and difficulties in properly clearing the unreacted cross-linking agents. Likewise, this method usually produces small-sized nanoparticles [38]. Other limitations associated with this technique include the need for organic solvents, a drawn-out procedure, and a difficult washing stage [39]. In this process, cross-linking chemicals like glutaraldehyde, sulfuric acid, and heat treatment are frequently used. The preparation and functionality of the microspheres can also be impacted by the chitosan and stabilizing solution concentrations. The method has been effectively used to encapsulate a number of medications, including diclofenac sodium, phenobarbital, nifedipine, theophylline, griseofulvin, pentazocine, progesterone, and others, despite these limitations.

2.2.2 Ionotropic gelation method

Because of the limitations of emulsion cross-linking procedures, there has been increased interest in the formation of complexes of macromolecules characterized by opposite charges to produce chitosan microspheres. This method, known as ionic gelation, provides a simple and gentle technique that eliminates the need for harsh cross-linking chemicals. Through electrostatic forces, tripolyphosphate (TPP), a polyanion, interacts with the cationic chitosan. The chitosan is dispersed in an acidic solution to get the cationic form. This solution is then dropped into a TPP solution while being stirred. Ionic gelation occurs as a result of the complexation of oppositely charged species, resulting in the creation of spherical particles. TPP/chitosan microparticles, on the other hand, have low mechanical strength, limiting their applicability in drug delivery applications. The ionotropic gelation method has several advantages, including gentle processing conditions, the utilization of an aqueous medium, low toxicity, and minimum drug chemical modification. However, it has limitations such as low acidic stability and difficulty in encapsulating high molecular weight drugs [39, 40].

For the production of protein-loaded CS, an altered ionotropic gelation process utilizing a high voltage electrostatic field was developed. As a model protein, bovine serum albumin (BSA) was used [41]. When a solution of sodium tripolyphosphate (TPP) and ethanol was utilized as the coagulation solution, the microspheres showed good sphericity and dispersity. For BSA-to-chitosan weight ratios less than 5%, encapsulation efficiency was greater than 90%. The amount of BSA liberated from the microspheres varied according to the coagulation solution and pH. At pH 8.8, around 35% of BSA was relinquished from microspheres cured in a 3% coagulation solution, while over 50% was liberated from microspheres cured in a 1% coagulation solution. In a 1% coagulation solution at pH 4, only 15% of the BSA was released. The findings show that combining ionotropic gelation with a high voltage electrostatic field is an efficient way for producing chitosan microspheres for long-term protein administration. Furthermore, chitosan microspheres produced via tripolyphosphate cross-linking and emulsification ionotropic gelation have been demonstrated to be an efficient mucoadhesive delivery strategy [5].

2.2.3 Coacervation/precipitation approach

This approach is based on the distinct physicochemical features of chitosan. Because chitosan is insoluble in alkaline solutions, upon exposure to them, it produces precipitates or coacervates. Using a compressed air nozzle, a chitosan solution is sprayed into an alkali solution, such as sodium hydroxide, NaOH-methanol, or ethanediamine. The particles are then separated by filtration or centrifugation and rinsed with heated and chilled water. Particle size may be regulated by altering compressed air pressure or spray-nozzle diameter, while drug release can be controlled by utilizing cross-linking agents. DNA-chitosan nanoparticles can be created via the coacervation of positively charged chitosan amine groups and negatively charged DNA phosphate groups [42, 43]. This approach has some limitations, such as poor nanoparticle stability, limited drug loading, and the requirement for complex cross-linking using chemical agents such as toxic glutaraldehyde [44, 45].

The Polyelectrolyte Complex (PEC) approach, on the contrary, includes mechanically swirling at room temperature of an anionic solution such as dextran sulfate DNA solution into a cationic polymer solution like chitosan solution dissolved in acetic acid, gelatin, or polyethylenimine. As a result, charge neutralization occurs, and nanoparticles are formed. The PEC approach has various advantages, including its simplicity, moderate conditions, and the creation of spontaneous nanoparticles [39, 44]. For example, insulin-loaded chitosan nanoparticles having a mean diameter of around 200 nm and a sustained *in vitro* release profile were created utilizing the PEC approach with low molecular weight water-soluble chitosan (LMWSC) nanoparticles [44]. This process of chitosan microspheres is further demonstrated in **Figure 2**.

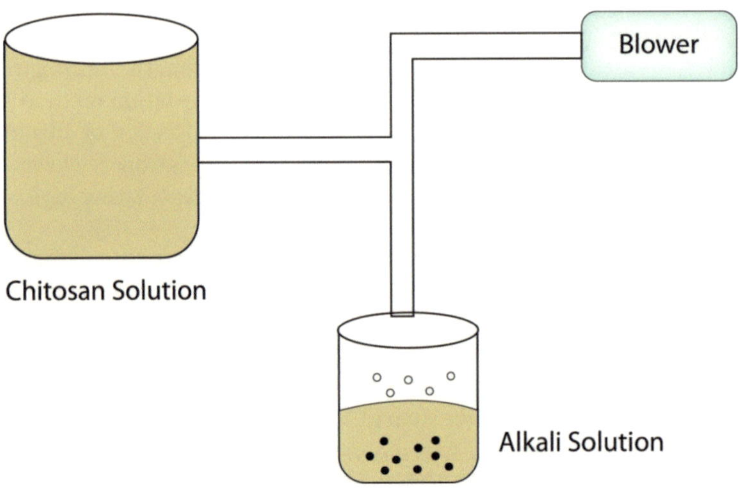

Figure 2.
Representing the preparation of chitosan microspheres by coacervation/precipitation. In this method, a chitosan solution is sprayed into an alkaline solution through a nozzle that uses compressed air, which results in the formation of tiny droplets known as coacervates. Afterward, these particles are collected and cleaned through methods such as filtration or centrifugation. This is followed by a series of washes with both hot and cold water to ensure thorough purification. Figure was adopted and redesigned from the work of Garg et al. [46].

2.2.4 Emulsion-droplet coalescence method

Tokumitsu et al. created a novel emulsion-droplet coalescence technique that combines both emulsion cross-linking and precipitation principles [47]. Instead of cross-linking stable droplets, this approach initiates precipitation by combining chitosan and NaOH droplets. The procedure includes the formation of two stable emulsions: one having an aqueous solution of chitosan and the medication, and the other containing an aqueous solution of chitosan and NaOH. When these emulsions are aggressively combined, the droplets from each emulsion collide and fuse, causing chitosan droplets to precipitate, and tiny particles are formed. This method was employed to create gadopentetic acid-loaded chitosan nanoparticles for gadolinium neutron-capture therapy. Notably, no cross-linking agent is used in this approach, which may block the unbound amino groups of chitosan; instead, the connection between gadopentetic acid (a bivalent anionic molecule) and the amino groups of chitosan is based on electrostatic forces. Nanomaterials with an average particle size of 452 nm and a drug loading capacity of 45% were successfully synthesized using 100% deacetylated chitosan under the emulsion-droplet coalescence process. This method permitted increased gadopentetic acid loading in comparison to the simple emulsion cross-linking method [5]. This method of preparation of chitosan microparticles is further demonstrated in **Figure 3**.

2.2.5 Reverse micellar approach

In this approach, the surfactant is disseminated in an organic solvent resulting in the formation of reverse micelles, which are liquid mixes of water, oil, as well as surfactant.

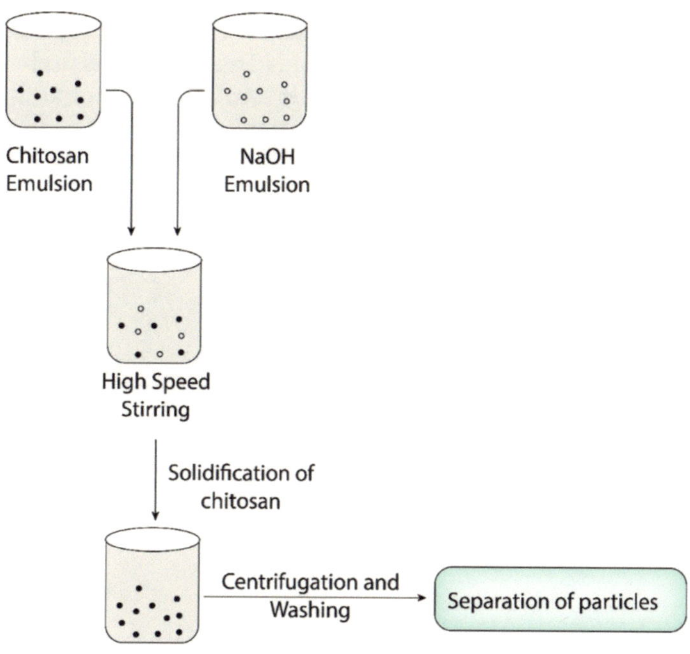

Figure 3.
Diagrammatic representation of preparation of chitosan nanoparticles by emulsion-droplet coalescence method. Figure was adopted and redesigned from the work of Garg et al. [46].

Aqueous solutions consisting of chitosan and the drug are delivered into the reverse micelles with continuous vortexing to retain optical clarity and generate a microemulsion. Controlling the water concentration in the aqueous phase precisely is critical to ensuring that the entire combination stays optically clear. More water can be added if bigger nanoparticles are needed. After achieving a clear solution, a cross-linking agent is introduced with consistent mixing, and the cross-linking reaction is then allowed to occur overnight. The utmost quantity of the drug that can be disseminated in the reverse micelles is ascertained by steadily increasing the drug concentration until the clear microemulsion turns into a translucent solution. The organic solvent subsequently evaporates, leaving an apparent dry material. When a suitable amount of salt is included to this substance, it causes the surfactant to precipitate from the solution. The mixture is centrifuged, and the supernatant solution that results includes the drug-loaded nanoparticles. To remove impurities and unbound pharmaceuticals, the aqueous dispersion is dialyzed for roughly 1 h using a dialysis membrane. Finally, the residual liquid is lyophilized, yielding chitosan nanoparticles in dry powder form. The approach leverages reverse micelles and microemulsion systems to create chitosan nanoparticles, allowing for regulated drug encapsulation inside nanoparticles and thus offering a diverse strategy for drug delivery applications [5, 48]. This process of preparing chitosan microparticles is diagrammatically shown in **Figure 4**.

2.2.6 Sieving method

Agnihotri and Aminabhavi described a simple and emerging approach for generating CMs carrying the drug clozapine [49]. The procedure begins with the dissolution of a certain amount of chitosan in a 4% acetic acid solution, which results in the production of a thick, gel-like material. This mass is then subsequently cross-linked using glutaraldehyde, changing it into a non-adhesive, cross-linked substance. This substance is then put through a sieve with a suitable mesh size to yield microparticles. Following that, the microparticles are then washed with 0.1 N NaOH solutions to eliminate any leftover glutaraldehyde before drying overnight in a 40°C oven. Prior to cross-linking, the drug clozapine is incorporated into chitosan, resulting in an impressive encapsulation efficacy of up to 98.9%. This approach has the benefit of being simple and

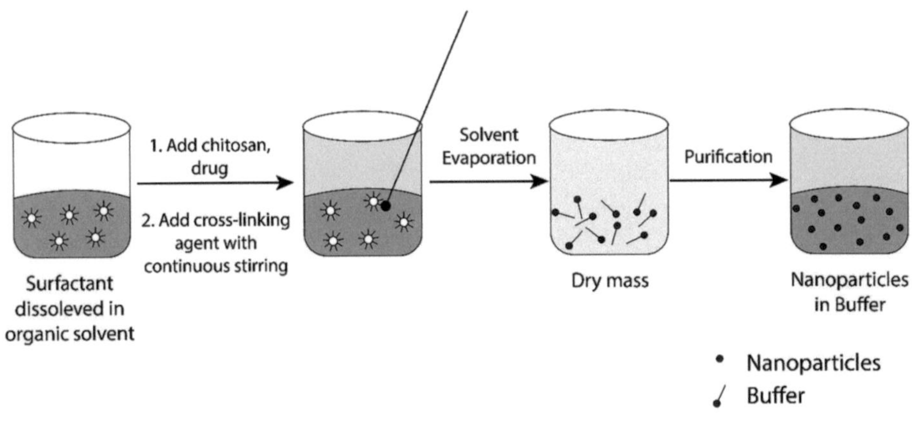

Figure 4.
Diagrammatic representation of chitosan nanoparticles preparation by reverse micellar method. Figure was adopted and redesigned from the work of Garg et al. [46].

scalable, as it eliminates the need for sophisticated operations. The generated microparticles, however, were of various forms, with average particle sizes ranging from 543 to 698 μm. *In vitro* studies revealed that clozapine may be released over a 12-hour period, however, *in vivo* studies revealed a slower drug release profile [5].

2.2.7 Solvent evaporation approach

This approach is based on the formation of an emulsion from a polymer solution with either a nonaqueous (water-in-oil) or an aqueous (oil-in-water) continuous phase. A solvent, such as liquid paraffin or acetone, is utilized in this procedure.

The requisite molecule is first dissolved in acetone and then disseminated in a chitosan solution. This combination is emulsified into liquid paraffin with constant agitation. The resultant microsphere suspension is filtered, washed, and dried to produce the desired particle size. To prevent clumping, magnesium stearate is frequently introduced during the preparation process as an anti-agglomeration agent. Interestingly, increasing the amount of magnesium stearate employed in the procedure tends to reduce the average particle size [50].

2.2.8 Spray drying approach

Spray drying is another well-known method for producing chitosan microspheres (CMs). In this method, a chitosan solution is aerosolized and subjected to air-drying, then a cross-linking agent is introduced. He et al. used various emulsions, notably oil-in-water-in-oil or water-in-oil-in-water emulsions, to generate CMs for spray drying cimetidine and famotidine encapsulation. When compared to microspheres produced via standard spray drying or the oil-in-water emulsion approach, the resultant microspheres demonstrated a comparatively sustained and regulated drug release [50, 51]. Using this approach, the chitosan microspheres can be manufactured in a variety of forms to improve their specific features and ensure optimal drug delivery. Below, we shall discuss some of the types of chitosan microspheres and their potential applications in drug delivery.

2.2.8.1 Mucoadhesive microspheres

Mucoadhesive property pertains to a substance's capacity, in this context, microspheres or other drug delivery systems, to cling or stick to the mucosal surfaces of biological tissues, which include those found in the respiratory, gastrointestinal, or nasal tracts. This characteristic enables the material to remain in touch with the mucosal barrier for a prolonged length of time, improving its efficacy for delivering drug or vaccine administration. Microspheres with mucoadhesive qualities have significant advantages, including the ability to extend residence duration and increase vaccination absorption when added to them. Mucoadhesive drug delivery methods have been shown to improve drug bioavailability, increase macromolecule absorption, and extend residence duration at the application site [52].

One of the most important aspects of microparticles in vaccine delivery is their capacity to acquire an appropriate size for effective trafficking inside the body and uptake by antigen-presenting cells (APCs). Drug-loaded microspheres of suitable size have been shown in studies to be absorbed by APCs, enabling vaccine delivery across cell membranes [53]. The size of microparticles is a crucial factor in immunogenicity, with smaller particles (<10 μm) typically more immune-stimulating than bigger ones

(>10 μm) [54, 55]. Microspheres also have the advantage of extending the residence period of vaccinations at mucosal surfaces as compared to solutions. Microspheres have been shown to have an immediate impact on nasal mucosa by dehydrating epithelial cells, inducing tight junctions to separate imbibing water from mucus and swell [56]. The extended habitation period of microspheres at mucosal surfaces can improve the uptake of vaccine formulations encapsulated with microspheres because of the extended contact between the vaccine and the mucosal membrane. Chitosan is the most frequently utilized natural polymer with possible applications in mucosal vaccination administration, among other mucoadhesive agents. Research is done to assess the role of chitosan microspheres in oral vaccination. In one study, Tian et al. found that fish vaccinated with chitosan microspheres containing plasmid DNA (pDNA) encoding the major capsid protein (MCP) gene of lymphocystis disease virus (LCDV) had significantly higher systemic immune responses than those vaccinated simply with pDNA [57].

2.2.8.2 Chitosan microspheres with Pluronics® F127

Chitosan microspheres, employed for regulated drug release and enhanced adjuvanticity, were developed in combination with Pluronic F127® (also referred to as F127), which acted as both a stabilizing as well as an immunomodulating agent [13]. Pluronics, also referred to as Poloxamers, are copolymers composed of poly(ethylene oxide) (PEO) and poly(propylene oxide) (PPO) (PEO-b-PPO-b-PEO), and are widely used in pharmaceutical applications. These compounds function as flexible pharmacological excipients, enhancing drugs solubility and stability in aqueous conditions [58]. F127 has received extensive interest as a temperature-responsive material owing to its remarkable thermo-reversible gelation capabilities. It exhibits water solubility as well as excellent drug-release properties making it a good choice for drug delivery systems [59]. Numerous studies have looked at the usage of CS and F127 together as a vaccine delivery system. Intranasal vaccination with an antigen in F127/CS, for example, significantly elevated systemic and mucosal immune responses in comparison to control groups [60]. This improvement in immune responses was attributed to F127's capacity to stabilize the protein antigen, implying a synergistic impact between the two components. Another study found that intraperitoneal or subcutaneous injection of F127/CpG and F127/CS mixtures significantly increased antigen-specific systemic antibody responses in comparison to antigens combined with CpGs or chitosan alone [61]. The evidence suggests that F127 can work in tandem with chitosan and other immunomodulating drugs to increase the adjuvant effect. Adjuvants blend and drug delivery methods with distinct mechanisms of action have the potential to maximize immune responses.

2.2.8.3 Mannosylated chitosan microspheres

Antigen mannosylation is another potential approach to increase antigen immunogenicity via mannose receptor (MR) targeting present on professional antigen-presenting cells (APCs). Membrane-bound C-type lectin receptors, such as macrophage MRs (MMR, CD206), dendritic cell-specific intracellular adhesion molecule-3-grabbing nonintegrin (DC-SIGN, CD209), dectin-1, and langerin, have cytoplasmic tails with sorting motifs causing immediate uptake into clathrin-coated vesicles [62]. As a result, mannosylated antigens are absorbed by cells expressing these receptors, endocytosed, and transported to the acidic environment of early endosomes.

Mannosylation of antigens can dramatically improve T cell stimulation, with studies demonstrating a 100-fold increase in T cell-stimulating efficacy via mannose-binding receptors [63]. Mannose-mediated antigen absorption, in particular, results in 100- to 10,000-fold increased efficacy in activating MHC class II-restricted T lymphocytes [62, 63]. Mannosylated antigens are effectively internalized through the Dendritic Cells (DCs) which are subsequently positioned within MHC class II-specific compartments and lysosomes, which results in significantly greater efficacy in activating particular MHC class II-restricted T lymphocytes. Moreover, mannosylated drug delivery systems, such as mannosylated liposomes [64] and niosomes [65], demonstrate enhanced immunogenicity by targeting MRs in APCs.

Mannosylated chitosan or chitosan nano/microparticles are also being studied as receptor-mediated gene delivery methods [66, 67]. Hashimoto et al., for example, found that mannosylated chitosan is an effective gene delivery strategy with greater transfection potential and minimal cytotoxicity in macrophages. This approach includes the identification of mannose residues and associated receptors in the recognition of plasmid DNA/mannosylated chitosan complexes [66]. Another study found that mannosylated chitosan nanoparticles successfully delivered the IL-12 gene to dendritic cells within tumors, increasing anticancer immune responses [68]. This method, which involved intratumoral injection of mannosylated chitosan nanoparticle/plasmid encoding murine IL-12 complexes, resulted in considerable inhibition of tumor development, angiogenesis, cell cycle arrest, and apoptosis.

2.3 Drug delivery mechanism in chitosan microspheres

Several factors influence the release of therapeutic agents from CMs, including the degree of cross-linking, the structure, dimensions, and density of the particle framework, the physicochemical characteristics of the pharmaceutical compound, and the presence of adjunct agents. In addition, the *in vitro* release pattern is affected by pH, polarity, and enzyme availability in the dissolution medium [69]. The drug discharge from CMs occurs via three distinct pathways: (a) the release of drug from the particle exterior, (b) the diffusion of drug molecules traversing the engorged elastic matrix, and (c) the discharge of the drug due to polymer attrition. In instances where drug liberation occurs from the surface, the absorbed drug entities disintegrate quickly upon contact with the release media. A similar process directs the release of drugs trapped in the particle surface layer. This method of releasing drugs produces a noticeable burst effect. He et al. discovered that chitosan microspheres containing cimetidine exhibit this burst action during the earliest phases of disintegration [51]. When microspheres are formed using the spray drying approach, a significant portion of the medication is liberated within a few minutes. However, increasing the density of cross-linking can help reduce the burst release. The drug is released by diffusion in three stages. To begin with, water permeates the particle system, causing the matrix to inflate. Following that, the glassy polymer transforms into a rubbery matrix, and the third step involves drug diffusion from the swelling rubbery matrix. As a result, the drug is released gradually at first, then at a faster pace. This process is more visible, especially in the context of hydrogels. Kweon and Kang developed a chitosan-polyvinyl alcohol (PVA) matrix to study prednisolone release under various situations [70]. The relationship between drug release magnitude and square root of time was linear, showing diffusional release control. The degree of PVA grafting, heat treatment, or cross-link density was shown to impact drug release, while the effect of pH was less significant when compared to unmodified chitosan. Agnihotri

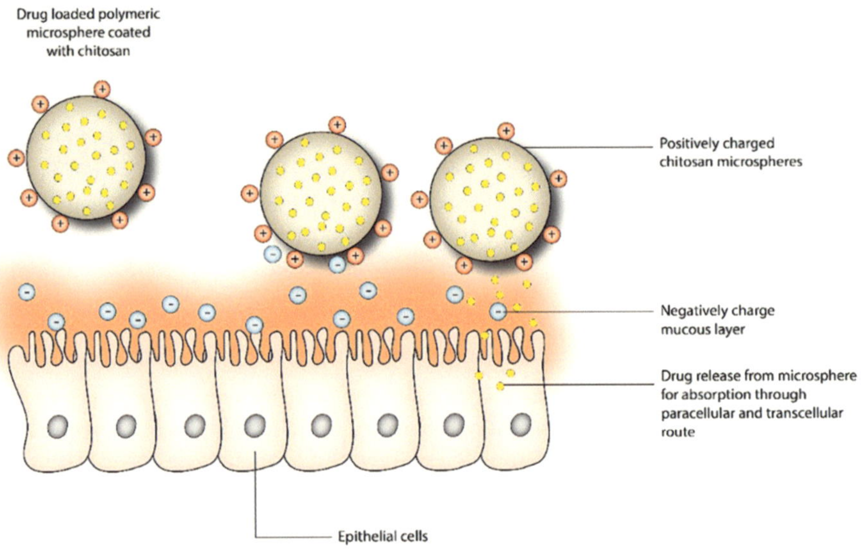

Figure 5.
Process of drug release from the chitosan microspheres. Figure was adopted and modified from the work of Mohammed et al. [15].

and Aminabhavi used the water absorption patterns of microparticles cross-linked with glutaraldehyde to examine the temporal changes in CMs swelling as a technique to predict drug release [49]. Notably, increased amounts of cross-linking resulted in less swelling of chitosan microparticles. Ameela et al. [12] discovered an association between cumulative drug liberation and the square root of time, confirming that drug release from the microsphere matrix is regulated by diffusion and follows the Higuchi equation [71]. Furthermore, the rate of liberation was determined to be dependent on the size of the microspheres. Orienti et al. investigated the relationship between matrix degradation and drug release kinetics in indomethacin-loaded chitosan microspheres [72]. The chitosan content within the microspheres and the pH of the release media were shown to be interdependent in the release kinetics. Notably, at high chitosan concentrations and at a pH of 7.4, deviations from Fick's law to zero-order kinetics were observed. **Figure 5** demonstrates the process of drug release from chitosan microspheres and absorption of the released drug through the paracellular and transcellular route. In the following few sections, we will explore some of the most important uses of CMs in drug delivery.

3. Applications of chitosan microspheres in drug delivery

Chitosan microspheres have a wide range of uses in novel drug delivery systems. Several of these applications are discussed below.

3.1 Applications of chitosan microspheres in nasal vaccines

Numerous studies have been conducted to investigate the use of chitosan microspheres as a delivery system for nasal vaccination. Van der Lubben et al. revealed that combining diphtheria toxoid with chitosan microparticles resulted in a considerable increase in IgG production following intranasal (IN) treatment. The rise in IgA responses, however, did not show a significant distinction from the control group [73]. Another notable observation was that bovine serum albumin (BSA) encapsulated inside chitosan microspheres caused higher antigen-specific IgG responses following IN vaccination compared to free BSA in solution [8]. Another study evaluated chitosan microspheres as a delivery mechanism for nasal immunization using mice and pigs [74]. Following IN injection of the antigen-loaded CMs, IgA antibody levels against the *Bordetella bronchiseptica* antigens in inoculated mice nasal washes elevated in a time- and dose-dependent manner [74]. Furthermore, antigen-specific IgA titers in nasal washes as well as saliva of pigs given the vaccine formulation via nasal vaccination showed a steady rise over time. Interestingly, the increased mucosal immune-stimulating effects of *Bordetella bronchiseptica*-loaded chitosan microspheres in both mice and pigs were accompanied by the induction of antigen-specific IgG antibody reactions in sera following identical vaccination regimens. Some studies have shown simultaneous use of a vaccine delivery technology and a mucosal adjuvant to synergistically improve immune responses in order to facilitate the development of more efficient mucosal vaccines. Following IN administration to mice, Baudner et al. found that a vaccine developed with chitosan microparticles along with a non-toxic LTK63 mutant of the heat-labile toxin (LT) caused higher levels of antigen-specific IgG in sera and antigen-specific IgA in nasal washes [14]. Using the same vaccination strategy, the researchers also explored another delivery system incorporating N-trimethyl chitosan microparticles. Mice inoculated intranasally with the vaccine containing N-trimethyl chitosan microparticles along with the LTK63 mutant exhibited higher levels of antigen-specific antibodies in their nasal washes, vaginal washes, and sera [14].

3.2 Applications of chitosan microspheres in oral delivery

Oral vaccine delivery has several advantages over traditional needle injections and is widely acknowledged as a reliable technique of immunization. However, injection-based vaccine administration still remains the most common method, owing to the lack of an adequate delivery route capable of reaching the target site of induction and increasing effector responses. Regardless of its likely preference as an alternative for vaccine administration, particularly in pediatric patients, oral delivery is hampered by antigen degradation within the gastrointestinal tract as well as displays inefficient localization at the intended site of action once administered in an unformulated state [50, 75]. As a result, the development of an effective delivery mechanism has been designated as the primary need in the field of oral vaccination. To elicit significant immune responses after oral administration, the vaccine must successfully reach M-cells in the Peyer's patches of the intestinal tract while avoiding the severe acidic pH environment of the stomach and enzymatic breakdown. Even when the vaccine comes extremely close to the Peyer's patches, immunological responses are not always triggered. This is mostly owing to the antigen access constraints to the Peyer's patches and ineffective absorption at the induction site. Researchers have found that incorporating vaccines with chitosan microspheres (CMs) significantly increases M-cell uptake and acts as a protective barrier against protein and peptide vaccine breakdown in the gastrointestinal tract [76–80]. Chitosan has thus been identified as a highly promising technique for oral vaccination due to its non-toxic nature and strong antigen-binding characteristics. Van der Lubben and colleagues [79, 80] have persistently conducted in-depth studies on CMs for mucosal vaccine administration, especially their absorption inside murine Peyer's patches, both *in vitro* and *in vivo*. A human intestinal M-cell model was methodically established by co-cultivating Caco-2 and Raji cells, allowing for a thorough analysis into CM uptake. This model, in particular, demonstrated no obvious structural alterations in the cellular monolayer and was useful in examining *in vitro* CM absorption for oral vaccine administration. The results proved unequivocally that CMs may be internalized by the epithelial lining of Peyer's patches [80]. Additionally, it has been determined that microparticles should preferably have diameters less than 10 μm in order to allow effective absorption by M-cells and access to the dome of Peyer's patches [81]. The CMs used in this study were much smaller than 10 μm, making them susceptible to M-cell absorption. Furthermore, due to chitosan's intrinsic biodegradability, van der Lubben et al. proposed that antigens get released from CMs following their absorption by M-cells [75, 80].

3.3 Applications of chitosan microspheres in GI delivery systems

Floating systems are distinguished by having a density lower than that of gastric juice. As a result, they increase the gastric residence time, consequently enhancing the bioavailability of drugs absorbed through the upper GI tract. Chitosan granules as well as chitosan-laminated preparations both have shown promising potential for the development of drug delivery methods that aim to reduce the influence of gastrointestinal transit time. Notably, the development of floating hollow microcapsules containing melatonin has resulted in an exciting gastroretentive controlled-release delivery method for drugs [50].

3.4 Chitosan microspheres in colonic and intestinal drug delivery

Chitosan microspheres are important in drug delivery to the colon and intestines. Chitosan is susceptible to breakdown by colonic bacteria, making it an attractive option for colon-specific medication delivery systems. Notably, chitosan esters like chitosan succinate and chitosan phthalate are shown to be useful as matrices for the colon-specific oral administration of drugs such as diclofenac sodium. With intriguing findings, researchers have also investigated systems for colon administration of drugs like paracetamol, mesalazine, and insulin. Establishing prolonged intestinal drug delivery for substances such as 5-fluorouracil (a treatment option for colon cancer) and insulin (a treatment option for diabetes mellitus) looks to serve as a viable substitute for injection therapy. To achieve this objective, formulations that avoid the acidic environment of the stomach and liberate the loaded drug over longer periods of time within the intestine have been developed. The bioadhesive characteristics of polyacrylic acid, alginate, and chitosan are mostly used in these formulations [5, 82, 83].

3.5 Chitosan microspheres in opthalmic drug delivery

In the realm of developing delivery systems for ocular drug administration, chitosan stands out as a special material. Ophthalmic chitosan gels demonstrate outstanding adhesion qualities to mucin, which creates a protective coating on the conjunctiva and corneal surface of the eye due to their remarkable elasticity.

Colloidal systems based on chitosan have shown to be excellent drug carriers via the mucosal route. These systems, such as chitosan-coated colloidal systems containing indomethacin, improve drug delivery to the inner eye. Furthermore, as revealed by chitosan nanoparticulate formulations containing cyclosporin, they allow drug accumulation within the corneal and conjunctival epithelia. Likewise, microparticulate drug carriers, especially microspheres, offer a potential strategy for topical acyclovir delivery to the eye [5, 84].

3.6 Chitosan microspheres in vaginal drug delivery

Vaginal pills incorporating chitosan, metronidazole, acriflavine, and other medications have shown efficient drug release, therapeutic effectiveness, and strong adhesion qualities. The addition of thiol groups to the polymer significantly improved its mucoadhesive characteristics, resulting in longer drug residency inside the vaginal mucosal tissue. This advancement provides regulated drug release, which is especially important in the treatment of mycotic infections, and improves therapeutic results [5, 49].

3.7 Chitosan microspheres in gene delivery system

Gene delivery has the potential to treat a wide range of hereditary disorders and multi-genetic diseases. Viral vectors, cationic liposomes, polycation complexes, as well as microencapsulated systems are examples of gene delivery systems. In these gene delivery applications, chitosan has emerged as a DNA carrier [5, 85]. Furthermore, because of its adhesive qualities and ability to facilitate gene transport across the gastrointestinal system, chitosan has the potential to be used as an oral gene carrier. Using chitosan and depolymerized chitosan oligomers, MacLaughlin et al. revealed *in vivo* the transport of plasmid DNA containing a cytomegalovirus (CMV) promoter sequence as well as a luciferase reporter gene, causing luciferase gene expression within the intestinal tract [86].

4. Limitations of CMs

Despite the various benefits of chitosan microspheres (CMs), such as biodegradability, non-toxicity, the ability to increase permeability, and the ability to crack tight junctions between epithelial cells, certain limitations do exist to their use. Various researchers have used CMs for vaccine delivery, and they discovered that vaccine-loaded CMs self-aggregated about 2 weeks following production [13, 87–90]. However, following nasal administration, these CMs remained efficient in generating immunological responses, including cytokine production *in vitro* and antigen-specific IgG and IgA responses *in vivo* [60, 88]. To avoid self-aggregation and improve stability, they included Pluronic F127 (F127) into the formulation to develop F127/CMs. These F127/CMs had a spherical shape with no aggregation for a long length of time, which was attributed to F127's hydrophilic polyethylene oxide chains, which hindered CM self-aggregation. When compared to CMs alone, F127/CMs demonstrated considerably better immunological activity *in vitro* and *in vivo*, as well as possible protection against infection [60].

Other investigations have found that CMs are unstable in acidic conditions, particularly when developed via precipitation method. The acidic stability of CMs produced by sodium sulfate precipitation was found to be low. The introduction of sodium sulfate to chitosan acetic acid solution resulted in ionic neutralization of the positively charged amine groups of chitosan, leading to chitosan derivatives with low solubility [91]. Similarly, the subsequent addition of acid (which increased the proton concentration) shifted the equilibrium favoring chitosan solubilization and resulting in the dissolution of CMs [92]. In another case, tripolyphosphate was used to make chitosan beads laden with sulfadiazine, however, the beads lacked mechanical strength [93]. In summary, CMs do have limitations that may be addressed by improvements. Incorporating F127, for example, is a useful method for increasing CM stability and mechanical strength. Furthermore, structural chitosan changes, such as the usage of thiolated chitosan, may improve the stability and usefulness of CMs.

5. Conclusion

Chitosan microspheres (CMs) are a highly promising mechanism for vaccine administration, both orally and nasally. This study provides a thorough evaluation of several ways to develop CMs, providing insights into the development of more sophisticated and functionalized chitosan-based carrier systems. The study emphasizes the importance of establishing appropriate particle sizes when producing vaccine-loaded CMs, as this aspect has a significant impact on the effective transport of vaccines to mucosa-associated lymphoid tissue, permitting optimal immune activation. Moreover, the chapter explored that vaccine-loaded CMs can trigger systemic and local immune responses in a dose- and time-dependent manner. Chitosan and its particulate form have intrinsic properties such as non-toxicity, high bioavailability, mucoadhesiveness, and biodegradability, making it a viable contender for efficient vaccine delivery in the near future. Furthermore, the enhanced features of modified CMs like elevated mucoadhesivity, membrane permeability, stability, and controlled or extended release of encapsulated vaccines (e.g., TCMs) indicate that they have the potential to be effective vaccine carrier systems. Continued study and the capacity to alter chitosan offer the possibility of improving its structural and physicochemical characteristics, hence increasing the applications of CM systems in vaccine administration.

Acknowledgements

The authors sincerely appreciate Dr. Noreen Latief for her insightful suggestions that contributed to the technical enhancement of this chapter.

Conflict of interest

The authors declare no conflict of interest regarding the publication of this book chapter.

Author details

Faisal Khan[1], Aakif Khan[2], Zia Ur Rahman[2] and Numan Fazal[3*]

1 Centre of Excellence in Molecular Biology, University of the Punjab, Lahore, Pakistan

2 University Institute of Medical Laboratory Technology, The University of Lahore, Lahore, Pakistan

3 Department of Bioengineering, University of Engineering and Applied Sciences, Swat, Pakistan

*Address all correspondence to: numansaadi@yahoo.com

References

[1] Charman WN, Chan HK, Finnin BC, Charman SA. Drug delivery: A key factor in realising the full therapeutic potential of drugs. Drug Development Research. 1999;**46**(3-4):316-327

[2] Kopecek J. Smart and genetically engineered biomaterials and drug delivery systems. European Journal of Pharmaceutical Sciences. 2003;**20**(1):1-16

[3] Agnihotri SA, Mallikarjuna NN, Aminabhavi TM. Recent advances on chitosan-based micro- and nanoparticles in drug delivery. Journal of Controlled Release. 2004;**100**(1):5-28

[4] Kaş HS. Chitosan: Properties, preparations and application to microparticulate systems. Journal of Microencapsulation. 1997;**14**(6):689-711

[5] Mitra A, Dey B. Chitosan microspheres in novel drug delivery systems. Indian Journal of Pharmaceutical Sciences. 2011;**73**(4):355-366

[6] Letchford K, Burt H. A review of the formation and classification of amphiphilic block copolymer nanoparticulate structures: Micelles, nanospheres, nanocapsules and polymersomes. European Journal of Pharmaceutics and Biopharmaceutics. 2007;**65**(3):259-269

[7] Anton N, Benoit JP, Saulnier P. Design and production of nanoparticles formulated from nano-emulsion templates—A review. Journal of Controlled Release. 2008;**128**(3): 185-199

[8] Alpar HO, Somavarapu S, Atuah KN, Bramwell VW. Biodegradable mucoadhesive particulates for nasal and pulmonary antigen and DNA delivery. Advanced Drug Delivery Reviews. 2005;**57**(3):411-430

[9] Gavini E, Hegge AB, Rassu G, Sanna V, Testa C, Pirisino G, et al. Nasal administration of carbamazepine using chitosan microspheres: *In vitro*/*in vivo* studies. International Journal of Pharmaceutics. 2006;**307**(1):9-15

[10] Kang ML, Cho CS, Yoo HS. Application of chitosan microspheres for nasal delivery of vaccines. Biotechnology Advances. 2009;**27**(6):857-865

[11] Krauland AH, Guggi D, Bernkop-Schnürch A. Thiolated chitosan microparticles: A vehicle for nasal peptide drug delivery. International Journal of Pharmaceutics. 2006;**307**(2):270-277

[12] Lim S, Forbes B, Martin G, Brown M. *In vivo* and *in vitro* characterization of novel microparticulates based on hyaluronan and chitosan hydroglutamate. AAPS PharmSciTech. 2015;**2**(4):20

[13] Kang ML, Jiang HL, Kang SG, Guo DD, Lee DY, Cho CS, et al. Pluronic® F127 enhances the effect as an adjuvant of chitosan microspheres in the intranasal delivery of Bordetella bronchiseptica antigens containing dermonecrotoxin. Vaccine. 2007;**25**(23):4602-4610

[14] Baudner BC, Giuliani MM, Verhoef JC, Rappuoli R, Junginger HE, Giudice GD. The concomitant use of the LTK63 mucosal adjuvant and of chitosan-based delivery system enhances the immunogenicity and efficacy of intranasally administered vaccines. Vaccine. 2003;**21**(25):3837-3844

[15] Mohammed MA, Syeda JTM, Wasan KM, Wasan EK. An overview of chitosan nanoparticles and its application in non-parenteral drug delivery. Pharmaceutics. 2017;**9**(4):53

[16] Vårum KM, Ottøy MH, Smidsrød O. Water-solubility of partially N-acetylated chitosans as a function of pH: Effect of chemical composition and depolymerisation. Carbohydrate Polymers. 1994;**25**(2):65-70

[17] Borchard G, Lueβen HL, de Boer AG, Verhoef JC, Lehr CM, Junginger HE. The potential of mucoadhesive polymers in enhancing intestinal peptide drug absorption. III: Effects of chitosan-glutamate and carbomer on epithelial tight junctions *in vitro*. Journal of Controlled Release. 1996;**39**(2):131-138

[18] Dodane V, Amin Khan M, Merwin J. Effect of chitosan on epithelial permeability and structure. International Journal of Pharmaceutics. 1999;**182**(1):21-32

[19] Artursson P, Lindmark T, Davis SS, Illum L. Effect of chitosan on the permeability of monolayers of intestinal epithelial cells (Caco-2). Pharmaceutical Research. 1994;**11**(9):1358-1361

[20] Pan Y, Li Y, Zhao H, Zheng J, Xu H, Wei G, et al. Bioadhesive polysaccharide in protein delivery system: Chitosan nanoparticles improve the intestinal absorption of insulin *in vivo*. International Journal of Pharmaceutics. 2002;**249**(1):139-147

[21] Park SY, Jun ST, Marsh KS. Physical properties of PVOH/chitosan-blended films cast from different solvents. Food Hydrocolloids. 2001;**15**(4):499-502

[22] Mima S, Miya M, Iwamoto R, Yoshikawa S. Highly deacetylated chitosan and its properties. Journal of Applied Polymer Science. 1983;**28**(6):1909-1917

[23] Risbud MV, Hardikar AA, Bhat SV, Bhonde RR. pH-sensitive freeze-dried chitosan-polyvinyl pyrrolidone hydrogels as controlled release system for antibiotic delivery. Journal of Controlled Release. 2000;**68**(1):23-30

[24] Kolhe P, Kannan RM. Improvement in ductility of chitosan through blending and copolymerization with PEG: FTIR investigation of molecular interactions. Biomacromolecules. 2003;**4**(1):173-180

[25] Koul V, Mohamed R, Kuckling D, Adler HJP, Choudhary V. Interpenetrating polymer network (IPN) nanogels based on gelatin and poly(acrylic acid) by inverse miniemulsion technique: Synthesis and characterization. Colloids and Surfaces. B, Biointerfaces. 2011;**83**(2):204-213

[26] Elhefian E, Yahaya A. Rheological study of chitosan and its blends: An overview. Maejo International Journal of Science and Technology. 2010;**4**:210-220

[27] Shukla SK, Mishra AK, Arotiba OA, Mamba BB. Chitosan-based nanomaterials: A state-of-the-art review. International Journal of Biological Macromolecules. 2013;**59**:46-58

[28] Dambies L, Vincent T, Domard A, Guibal E. Preparation of chitosan gel beads by ionotropic molybdate gelation. Biomacromolecules. 2001;**2**(4):1198-1205

[29] Al-Qadi S, Grenha A, Carrión-Recio D, Seijo B, Remuñán-López C. Microencapsulated chitosan nanoparticles for pulmonary protein delivery: *in vivo* evaluation of insulin-loaded formulations. Journal of Controlled Release. 2012;**157**(3):383-390

[30] Thanou MM, Kotzé AF, Scharringhausen T, Luessen HL, de Boer AG, Verhoef JC, et al. Effect of degree of quaternization of N-trimethyl chitosan chloride for enhanced transport of hydrophilic compounds across intestinal caco-2 cell monolayers. Journal of Controlled Release. 2000;**64**(1-3):15-25

[31] Bernkop-Schnürch A, Hornof M, Zoidl T. Thiolated polymers--thiomers: Synthesis and *in vitro* evaluation of chitosan-2-iminothiolane conjugates. International Journal of Pharmaceutics. 2003;**260**(2):229-237

[32] Sadeghi AMM, Dorkoosh FA, Avadi MR, Weinhold M, Bayat A, Delie F, et al. Permeation enhancer effect of chitosan and chitosan derivatives: Comparison of formulations as soluble polymers and nanoparticulate systems on insulin absorption in Caco-2 cells. European Journal of Pharmaceutics and Biopharmaceutics. 2008;**70**(1):270-278

[33] Yin L, Ding J, He C, Cui L, Tang C, Yin C. Drug permeability and mucoadhesion properties of thiolated trimethyl chitosan nanoparticles in oral insulin delivery. Biomaterials. 2009;**30**(29):5691-5700

[34] Cui F, Qian F, Zhao Z, Yin L, Tang C, Yin C. Preparation, characterization, and oral delivery of insulin loaded carboxylated chitosan grafted poly(methyl methacrylate) nanoparticles. Biomacromolecules. 2009;**10**(5):1253-1258

[35] Kurita K, Hashimoto S, Yoshino H, Ishii S, Nishimura SI. Preparation of chitin/polystyrene hybrid materials by efficient graft copolymerization based on mercaptochitin. Macromolecules. 1996;**29**(6):1939-1942

[36] Furlani F, Sacco P, Marsich E, Donati I, Paoletti S. Highly monodisperse colloidal coacervates based on a bioactive lactose-modified chitosan: From synthesis to characterization. Carbohydrate Polymers. 2017;**174**:360-368

[37] Sacco P, Paoletti S, Cok M, Asaro F, Abrami M, Grassi M, et al. Insight into the ionotropic gelation of chitosan using tripolyphosphate and pyrophosphate as cross-linkers. International Journal of Biological Macromolecules. 2016;**92**:476-483

[38] Wang Y, Wang X, Luo G, Dai Y. Adsorption of bovin serum albumin (BSA) onto the magnetic chitosan nanoparticles prepared by a microemulsion system. Bioresource Technology. 2008;**99**(9):3881-3884

[39] Nagpal K, Singh SK, Mishra DN. Chitosan nanoparticles: A promising system in novel drug delivery. Chemical and Pharmaceutical Bulletin (Tokyo). 2010;**58**(11):1423-1430

[40] Gonçalves IC, Henriques PC, Seabra CL, Martins MCL. The potential utility of chitosan micro/nanoparticles in the treatment of gastric infection. Expert Review of Anti-Infective Therapy. 2014;**12**(8):981-992

[41] Shu XZ, Zhu KJ. A novel approach to prepare tripolyphosphate/chitosan complex beads for controlled release drug delivery. International Journal of Pharmaceutics. 2000;**201**(1):51-58

[42] Zhao K, Shi X, Zhao Y, Wei H, Sun Q, Huang T, et al. Preparation and immunological effectiveness of a swine influenza DNA vaccine encapsulated in chitosan nanoparticles. Vaccine. 2011;**29**(47):8549-8556

[43] Zhuo Y, Han J, Tang L, Liao N, Gui GF, Chai YQ, et al. Quenching of the emission of peroxydisulfate system by ferrocene functionalized

chitosan nanoparticles: A sensitive "signal off" electrochemiluminescence immunosensor. Sensors and Actuators B: Chemical. 2014;**192**:791-795

[44] Chandra Hembram K, Prabha S, Chandra R, Ahmed B, Nimesh S. Advances in preparation and characterization of chitosan nanoparticles for therapeutics. Artificial Cells, Nanomedicine, and Biotechnology. 2016;**44**(1):305-314

[45] Huang M, Fong CW, Khor E, Lim LY. Transfection efficiency of chitosan vectors: Effect of polymer molecular weight and degree of deacetylation. Journal of Controlled Release. 2005;**106**(3):391-406

[46] Garg U, Chauhan S, Nagaich U, Jain N. Current advances in chitosan nanoparticles based drug delivery and targeting. Advanced Pharmaceutical Bulletin. 2019;**9**(2):195-204

[47] Tokumitsu H, Ichikawa H, Fukumori Y. Chitosan-gadopentetic acid complex nanoparticles for gadolinium neutron-capture therapy of cancer: Preparation by novel emulsion-droplet coalescence technique and characterization. Pharmaceutical Research. 1999;**16**(12):1830-1835

[48] Mitra S, Gaur U, Ghosh PC, Maitra AN. Tumour targeted delivery of encapsulated dextran-doxorubicin conjugate using chitosan nanoparticles as carrier. Journal of Controlled Release. 2001;**74**(1-3):317-323

[49] Agnihotri SA, Aminabhavi TM. Controlled release of clozapine through chitosan microparticles prepared by a novel method. Journal of Controlled Release. 2004;**96**(2):245-259

[50] Islam MA, Firdous J, Choi YJ, Yun CH, Cho CS. Design and application of chitosan microspheres as oral and nasal vaccine carriers: An updated review. International Journal of Nanomedicine. 2012;**7**:6077-6093

[51] He P, Davis SS, Illum L. Chitosan microspheres prepared by spray drying. International Journal of Pharmaceutics. 1999;**187**(1):53-65

[52] Chowdary KPR, Rao YS. Mucoadhesive microspheres for controlled drug delivery. Biological and Pharmaceutical Bulletin. 2004;**27**(11):1717-1724

[53] Desai MP, Labhasetwar V, Walter E, Levy RJ, Amidon GL. The mechanism of uptake of biodegradable microparticles in Caco-2 cells is size dependent. Pharmaceutical Research. 1997;**14**(11):1568-1573

[54] Eldridge JH, Staas JK, Meulbroek JA, McGhee JR, Tice TR, Gilley RM. Biodegradable microspheres as a vaccine delivery system. Molecular Immunology. 1991;**28**(3):287-294

[55] Jeffery H, Davis SS, O'Hagan DT. The preparation and characterization of poly(lactide-co-glycolide) microparticles. II. The entrapment of a model protein using a (water-in-oil)-in-water emulsion solvent evaporation technique. Pharmaceutical Research. 1993;**10**(3):362-368

[56] Pereswetoff-Morath L. Microspheres as nasal drug delivery systems. Advanced Drug Delivery Reviews. 1998;**29**(1):185-194

[57] Tian J, Yu J, Sun X. Chitosan microspheres as candidate plasmid vaccine carrier for oral immunisation of Japanese flounder (*Paralichthys olivaceus*). Veterinary Immunology and Immunopathology. 2008;**126**(3):220-229

[58] Wang P, Johnston TP. Enhanced stability of two model proteins in

an agitated solution environment using poloxamer 407. PDA Journal of Pharmaceutical Science and Technology. 1993;**47**(4):183-189

[59] Agafonov M, Volkova T, Kumeev R, Chibunova E, Terekhova I. Impact of pluronic F127 on aqueous solubility and membrane permeability of antirheumatic compounds of different structure and polarity. Journal of Molecular Liquids. 2019;**274**:770-777

[60] Julie Westerink MA, Louise Smithson S, Srivastava N, Blonder J, Coeshott C, Rosenthal GJ. ProJuvant™ (Pluronic F127®/chitosan) enhances the immune response to intranasally administered tetanus toxoid. Vaccine. 2001;**20**(5):711-723

[61] Coeshott CM, Smithson SL, Verderber E, Samaniego A, Blonder JM, Rosenthal GJ, et al. Pluronic® F127-based systemic vaccine delivery systems. Vaccine. 2004;**22**(19):2396-2405

[62] Burudi EME, Régnier-Vigouroux A. Regional and cellular expression of the mannose receptor in the post-natal developing mouse brain. Cell and Tissue Research. 2001;**303**(3):307-317

[63] Engering AJ, Cella M, Fluitsma D, Brockhaus M, Hoefsmit ECM, Lanzavecchia A, et al. The mannose receptor functions as a high capacity and broad specificity antigen receptor in human dendritic cells. European Journal of Immunology. 1997;**27**(9):2417-2425

[64] Hattori Y, Kawakami S, Suzuki S, Yamashita F, Hashida M. Enhancement of immune responses by DNA vaccination through targeted gene delivery using mannosylated cationic liposome formulations following intravenous administration in mice. Biochemical and Biophysical Research Communications. 2004;**317**(4):992-999

[65] Gupta PN, Mishra V, Rawat A, Dubey P, Mahor S, Jain S, et al. Non-invasive vaccine delivery in transfersomes, niosomes and liposomes: A comparative study. International Journal of Pharmaceutics. 2005;**293**(1):73-82

[66] Hashimoto M, Morimoto M, Saimoto H, Shigemasa Y, Yanagie H, Eriguchi M, et al. Gene transfer by DNA/mannosylated chitosan complexes into mouse peritoneal macrophages. Biotechnology Letters. 2006;**28**(11):815-821

[67] Xing L, Fan YT, Zhou TJ, Gong JH, Cui LH, Cho KH, et al. Chemical modification of chitosan for efficient vaccine delivery. Molecules. 2018;**23**(2):229

[68] Kim TH, Jin H, Kim HW, Cho MH, Cho CS. Mannosylated chitosan nanoparticle–based cytokine gene therapy suppressed cancer growth in BALB/c mice bearing CT-26 carcinoma cells. Molecular Cancer Therapeutics. 2006;**5**(7):1723-1732

[69] Nam YS, Park TG. Protein loaded biodegradable microspheres based on PLGA-protein bioconjugates. Journal of Microencapsulation. 1999;**16**(5):625-637

[70] Kweon DK, Kang DW. Drug-release behavior of chitosan-g-poly(vinyl alcohol) copolymer matrix. Journal of Applied Polymer Science. 1999;**74**(2):458-464

[71] Higuchi T. Mechanism of sustained-action medication. Theoretical analysis of rate of release of solid drugs dispersed in solid matrices. Journal of Pharmaceutical Sciences. 1963;**52**:1145-1149

[72] Orienti I, Aiedeh K, Gianasi E, Ponti C, Zecchi V. Chitosan-

indomethacin conjugates. Effect of different substituents on the polysaccharide molecule on drug release. Archiv der Pharmazie. 1996;**329**(5):245-250

[73] van der Lubben IM, Kersten G, Fretz MM, Beuvery C, Coos Verhoef J, Junginger HE. Chitosan microparticles for mucosal vaccination against diphtheria: Oral and nasal efficacy studies in mice. Vaccine. 2003;**21**(13):1400-1408

[74] Kang ML, Kang SG, Jiang HL, Guo DD, Lee DY, Rayamahji N, et al. Chitosan microspheres containing Bordetella bronchiseptica antigens as novel vaccine against atrophic rhinitis in pigs. Journal of Microbiology and Biotechnology. 2008;**18**(6):1179-1185

[75] van der Lubben IM, Verhoef JC, van Aelst AC, Borchard G, Junginger HE. Chitosan microparticles for oral vaccination: Preparation, characterization and preliminary *in vivo* uptake studies in murine Peyer's patches. Biomaterials. 2001;**22**(7):687-694

[76] Bogataj M, Mrhar A, Grabnar I, Rajtman Z, Bukovec P, Srcic S, et al. The influence of magnesium stearate on the characteristics of mucoadhesive microspheres. Journal of Microencapsulation. 2000;**17**(4):499-508

[77] He P, Davis SS, Illum L. Sustained release chitosan microspheres prepared by novel spray drying methods. Journal of Microencapsulation. 1999;**16**(3):343-355

[78] Ozbaş-Turan S, Akbuğa J, Aral C. Controlled release of interleukin-2 from chitosan microspheres. Journal of Pharmaceutical Sciences. 2002;**91**(5):1245-1251

[79] Van Der Lubben IM, Konings FA, Borchard G, Verhoef JC, Junginger HE. *In vivo* uptake of chitosan microparticles by murine Peyer's patches: Visualization studies using confocal laser scanning microscopy and immunohistochemistry. Journal of Drug Targeting. 2001;**9**(1):39-47

[80] van der Lubben IM, van Opdorp FAC, Hengeveld MR, Onderwater JJM, Koerten HK, Verhoef JC, et al. Transport of chitosan microparticles for mucosal vaccine delivery in a human intestinal M-cell model. Journal of Drug Targeting. 2002;**10**(6):449-456

[81] Giudice EL, Campbell JD. Needle-free vaccine delivery. Advanced Drug Delivery Reviews. 2006;**58**(1):68-89

[82] Park HS, Lee JY, Cho SH, Baek HJ, Lee SJ. Colon delivery of prednisolone based on chitosan coated polysaccharide tablets. Archives of Pharmacal Research. 2002;**25**(6):964-968

[83] Tozaki H, Odoriba T, Okada N, Fujita T, Terabe A, Suzuki T, et al. Chitosan capsules for colon-specific drug delivery: Enhanced localization of 5-aminosalicylic acid in the large intestine accelerates healing of TNBS-induced colitis in rats. Journal of Controlled Release. 2002;**82**(1):51-61

[84] Genta I, Conti B, Perugini P, Pavanetto F, Spadaro A, Puglisi G. Bioadhesive microspheres for ophthalmic administration of acyclovir. The Journal of Pharmacy and Pharmacology. 1997;**49**(8):737-742

[85] Lee KY, Kwon IC, Kim YH, Jo WH, Jeong SY. Preparation of chitosan self-aggregates as a gene delivery system. Journal of Controlled Release. 1998;**51**(2-3):213-220

[86] MacLaughlin FC, Mumper RJ, Wang J, Tagliaferri JM, Gill I, Hinchcliffe M, et al. Chitosan and

depolymerized chitosan oligomers as condensing carriers for *in vivo* plasmid delivery. Journal of Controlled Release. 1998;**56**(1-3):259-272

[87] Jiang HL, Kang ML, Quan JS, Kang SG, Akaike T, Yoo HS, et al. The potential of mannosylated chitosan microspheres to target macrophage mannose receptors in an adjuvant-delivery system for intranasal immunization. Biomaterials. 2008;**29**(12):1931-1939

[88] Jiang HL, Park IK, Shin NR, Kang SG, Yoo HS, Kim SI, et al. *In vitro* study of the immune stimulating activity of an atrophic [correction of athrophic] rhinitis vaccine associated to chitosan microspheres. European Journal of Pharmaceutics and Biopharmaceutics. 2004;**58**(3):471-476

[89] Jiang HL, Park IK, Shin NR, Yoo HS, Akaike T, Cho CS. Controlled release of Bordetella bronchiseptica dermonecrotoxin (BBD) vaccine from BBD-loaded chitosan microspheres *in vitro*. Archives of Pharmacal Research. 2004;**27**(3):346-350

[90] Kang ML, Kang SG, Jiang HL, Shin SW, Lee DY, Ahn JM, et al. *In vivo* induction of mucosal immune responses by intranasal administration of chitosan microspheres containing Bordetella bronchiseptica DNT. European Journal of Pharmaceutics and Biopharmaceutics. 2006;**63**(2):215-220

[91] Berthold A, Cremer K, Kreuter J. Preparation and characterization of chitosan microspheres as drug carrier for prednisolone sodium phosphate as model for anti-inflammatory drugs. Journal of Controlled Release. 1996;**39**(1):17-25

[92] Illum L. Chitosan and its use as a pharmaceutical excipient. Pharmaceutical Research. 1998;**15**(9):1326-1331

[93] Bodmeier R, Oh KH, Pramar Y. Preparation and evaluation of drug-containing chitosan beads. Drug Development and Industrial Pharmacy. 1989;**15**(9):1475-1494